FOOD VALUES
Cholesterol and Fats

OTHER BOOKS IN THE FOOD VALUES SERIES

FOOD VALUES

Cholesterol and Fats

Leah Wallach

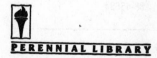

PERENNIAL LIBRARY

Harper & Row, Publishers, New York
Grand Rapids, Philadelphia, St. Louis, San Francisco
London, Singapore, Sydney, Tokyo, Toronto

Designed by Alma Orenstein

Library of Congress Cataloging-in-Publication Data

Wallach, Leah, 1947–
    Food values—cholesterol and fats.

    1. Food—Cholesterol content—Tables.   2. Food—Fat content—Tables.   I. Title.
TX553.C43W35   1989   641.1   88-45624
ISBN 0-06-096219-4

90 91 92 93 AG/BC 10 9 8 7 6 5 4 3

Contents

Foreword

By Robert E. Kowalski

The statistics are grim. Cardiovascular diseases claim one life in the United States every 32 seconds. Annually about 1,500,000 Americans suffer heart attacks; more than one-third of them die. Nearly a quarter of a million coronary bypass surgeries are performed each year. Ultimately nearly half of the population will die of some form of cardiovascular disease.

But such statistics do not entirely reveal the human dimensions of the nation's number one killer. Not particularly noted as a humanitarian, Joseph Stalin once said, "The death of one man is a tragedy; the death of one million is a statistic."

For the individuals and the families touched by heart disease, statistics don't mean much. The events are tragic.

A number of risk factors have been associated with heart disease, including family history, smoking, high blood pressure, a sedentary lifestyle, and stress. But none shows such a striking causative effect as elevated levels of cholesterol in the blood.

While the body requires a certain amount of cholesterol for vital functions such as the manufacture of cell walls, the production of hormones and bile acids used in digestion, and the formation of protective sheaths surrounding nerve cells, excessive levels begin to accumulate in the walls of arteries, gradually diminishing the flow of blood. In this process, called atherosclerosis, clogged arteries cannot supply sufficient blood to tissues including the heart, the brain, the legs, and other parts of the body. If the flow of blood ceases to provide oxygen to the heart, the result is myocardial infarction, otherwise known as heart attack.

Stop the flow of blood to the brain and you have a stroke. Impede the blood circulation in the legs and you have the sharp pain of intermittent claudication. And almost always the culprit is the same: cholesterol.

Dr. William Castelli, director of the famed Framingham Study, which investigated the correlation of certain factors with heart disease over decades in thousands of men, concluded that without excessive levels of cholesterol in the blood, coronary heart disease would be virtually unknown. He observed that he had never seen a heart attack in a man whose cholesterol level was under 155 milligrams per deciliter of blood (mg/dL). Others have noted that the incidence of heart attack climbs dramatically as cholesterol levels exceed a safety zone of from 160 to 180 mg/dL. And virtually every medical authority now agrees that every man and woman, regardless of age, should have a cholesterol level under 200.

Yet more than half the population has a level in excess of that 200 mg/dL maximum. No surprise, then, to learn that half the population will die of cardiovascular disease. More than a third will succumb to coronary heart disease alone. Though other risk factors contribute to the lethal picture, cholesterol remains a dominant component.

While the association between cholesterol levels in the blood and heart attacks and death was noted in the 1950s, a controversy raged for years as to whether changing the diet would or could have anything to do with the disease process. First, early dietary manipulations showed little if any impact on cholesterol levels in the blood. We've learned since then that both cholesterol and fat in the diet must be significantly reduced in order to lower cholesterol in the blood. Second, there was no proof that lowering those cholesterol levels could actually save lives. Finally that proof came in 1984 by way of the Lipid Research Clinic's Coronary Primary Prevention Trial, sponsored by the National Heart, Blood, and Lung Institute. Researchers found that for every 1% drop in cholesterol levels, there was a 2% decline in the risk of heart disease.

Armed with those and other data, which led to the conclusion that the need to reduce cholesterol levels in the population was urgent, the National Institutes of Health, along with twenty of the nation's major health organizations declared war on cholesterol. In a well-publicized press conference, authorities recommended that virtually all Americans should have their cholesterol levels tested, and that everyone, regardless of age or sex, should have a cholesterol level of no more than 200 mg/dL. Physicians were urged to test all patients. The public received education by way of the mass media and were encouraged to seek blood tests.

My own involvement began on a far more personal note. I have a family history of heart disease; my father had an elevated cholesterol level and died of a heart attack at 57 years of age. By the age of 41, I had suffered a heart attack and two bypass surgeries. Cholesterol was the culprit and something had to be done about it. The results of the program I developed were dramatic: within eight weeks my cholesterol level fell from a high of 284 to a very safe zone around 169. Others experienced similar reductions, and I then wrote *The 8-Week Cholesterol Cure* to share my findings.

Shortly thereafter, I learned that my son's cholesterol level was a bit high for his age. Nothing to be terribly worried about, but high enough so that if left to his own devices he'd grow up to have a level in the danger zone. I turned my attention to the area of cholesterol and children in the medical literature and found authorities agreeing that heart disease does, in fact, begin in childhood. It was time to change my son's eating habits. And my experiences were later shared in the book *Cholesterol and Children: A Parent's Guide to Giving Children a Future Free of Heart Disease*.

One fact emerges as being crystal clear: high levels of cholesterol in the blood put literally everyone at risk of heart disease and early death. This applies to men and women, boys and girls. The first step is to get a blood test. If the test indicates an elevation, it's time to do something about it. And the place to start is the diet.

Interestingly, though, heart disease is only one reason for modifying the diet. Data are rapidly accumulating which show convincingly that by reducing the fat content of the diet one can reduce the risk of cancer, diabetes, and obesity and can expect to live a longer life. Virtually every medical authority and organization recommend a significant reduction in fat and cholesterol intake.

The average American consumes about 40% of his or her calories as fat. Many of us eat a lot more than that. The American Heart Association has long stated that no one in the population should consume more than 30% of their calories as fat. The American Health Foundation brings that figure down to 20%. Nathan Pritikin advocated reductions to no more than 10%. I personally believe that a 20% to 25% level can be achieved without deprivation and will provide excellent results as part of a total program.

But how do you even know what your own percentage is? Most people have no idea what they're currently eating, much less how to reduce that level to any given percentage. I think percentages are far too abstract for the average person, including myself. So I show people how they can simplify the whole matter and at the same time tailor a dietary program for themselves. By doing so they never again have to count calories. Instead, they count the grams of fat and milligrams of cholesterol in the diet. The formulas for determining just how many grams of fat should be in your diet are found in this very helpful guide.

Once you know that magic number, you can proceed to choose a wide variety of delicious and nutritious foods from the major food groups. Now you can make food selections based on the amount of fat and cholesterol found in foods.

We hear a lot about cutting back on dairy foods, but what we really need to do is to cut back on the fat in those foods, not the foods themselves. That is to say, we need the nutrients from milk but not the fat. As you'll see in this guide, whole milk provides a whopping 8 or 9 grams of fat per serving. Switching to low-fat milk cuts that number in half. And by working down to skim milk, you virtually eliminate the fat. The trick is to do it gradually, so your taste buds can adjust. Today my children and I drink nothing but skim milk; the kids say "yuck" when given a glass of whole milk!

The same principles apply to meat. Eliminate red meat entirely? That's not necessary. Just learn which cuts have the least fat and opt for those lean varieties.

In terms of cutting back on cholesterol in the diet, just

remember that only animal foods contain that substance. There is no cholesterol, not even a tiny bit, in plant and vegetable foods. Thus when you hear that this peanut butter or that cooking oil contains no cholesterol, you know that it's just a matter of advertising hype: no oil or peanut butter contains any at all.

But some animal foods contain more cholesterol than others. Eggs and organ meats provide the most. Just look at the numbers. And while you're looking, you're in for a pleasant surprise in the shellfish department. Old techniques of testing indicated that shellfish were very high in cholesterol. That's because they were measuring all of the substances in the sterol family; only a portion of that total was cholesterol. Today we know that even shrimp can be enjoyed in moderation as part of a total dietary program. And some shellfish such as scallops are actually very low in cholesterol. This guide will show how to make wise choices, based on the latest information.

Some of those choices will be pretty obvious. We all know that butter is high in fat and cholesterol. But much of the fat in our diets is hidden in foods you might not think twice about before eating. And a lot of that fat is of the saturated type, the kind known to be the worst in terms of artery clogging.

We would never think of eating foods or beverages offered to us by a total stranger. We'd want to know what might be in those foods or drinks. Yet we think nothing of picking up foods in the market and eating them without any knowledge of what they might be made of.

Thus the first step toward becoming an informed consumer is to start reading the labels on foods. If you need a loaf of bread or some rolls, read the labels on a couple of brands. One might contain hydrogenated oils or coconut oil, while the other uses only soybean or corn oil as the shortening. You'll want to choose the latter.

If you're planning on a Mexican dinner, you should know that some refried beans and some flour tortillas are made with lard. Opt for the brands made with soybean oil. The labels will tell you which is which.

Don't be fooled by advertising ploys on the front of the package. A food that proclaims "No Cholesterol! Made Only with Vegetable Shortening!" might actually be laden with saturated fat in the form of coconut oil, palm oil, or palm kernel oil. Those tropical oils are actually more saturated, more artery clogging, than butter or lard.

The majority of processed foods today have a clearly stated nutrition label. Ingredients are listed in descending order by weight. And you'll see a breakdown of protein, carbohydrates, and fat in grams. Federal law mandates that any product making any health claim, such as "low in calories" or "reduced fat," must have a nutrition label.

But many foods don't have such labels. What about fresh meats, poultry, and seafood? What about baked goods? That's where this guide becomes particularly useful. You'll find all the information you need to make healthful choices.

You'll see that, whenever possible, the author has provided information about the amount of saturated fat in addition to the amount of total fat contained in a given food. Of the total fat in your diet, only one-third should come from saturated fats. In choosing between two foods, opt for the one with less saturated fat, even if both have the same amount of total fat.

This may all seem confusing at first, and perhaps even too complicated to deal with on a regular basis. Who has the time to do all that? you might complain. Trust me. Like anything else, learning about the fats and cholesterol in your diet will take a bit of time. But after a while it will be second nature. Today when my son Ross spots a new breakfast cereal, he checks to see if it contains coconut oil. My daughter Jenny, only 7 years old, knows she wants food without many grams of fat.

After just two or three trips to the supermarket, you'll know which breads, rolls, and other foods you want to buy routinely. As new foods appear on the market, check the labels. And become familiar with the data provided in this guide.

Is it all worth it? Only if you want to live a longer and healthier life!

Acknowledgments

I'd like to thank Laura Hickey, Shawn Connor, and Tim Bishop, who assisted me in the rather tedious task of entering data, and Alex Cantor, who typed and helped organize my correspondence with the food processors. I'd like also to acknowledge Helene A. Guthrie, whom I have never met but whose textbook, *Introductory Nutrition*, proved a most useful reference during the early stages of this project.

I'm grateful to all the scientists who allowed me to interview them in the course of preparing this book and particularly to Dr. DeWitt Goodman of Columbia University, Dr. Richard Rivlin and Dr. Martin Lipkin of Memorial Sloan-Kettering Cancer Center, Dr. Robert E. Olson of the School of Medicine, Health Sciences Center, the State University of New York at Stony Brook, and Dr. Dennis Ponton, chairman of the Nutrition and Food Science Department, Buffalo State College.

Introduction

Americans eat the equivalent of three-quarters of a cup of oil a day. Of course we don't swig a glass of the stuff. Some of the fat in our diet is a natural part of popular foods like hard cheeses and the beloved hamburger. We add fats and oil to other foods to flavor them: we make our chicken crisp by frying it in oil; we drench our muffins with butter or margarine, soak fresh salad in oils, plop sour cream on our baked potatoes, and serve fish reclining in melted butter.

Fats do make food more palatable and they should be a part of our diet—but not such a large part. Lipids, the generic term for fats, oils, and fatlike substances including cholesterol, now supply an average of 37% of the food energy—calories—in the American diet. The National Institutes of Health, the American Cancer Society, and the American Heart Association are confident that the incidence of coronary heart disease and possibly some cancers would be lowered if we reduced our fat intake to 30% of our total calories.

Fats and Oils

About 20% of the body weight of a healthy 25-year-old woman and 15% of the body weight of a healthy young man is fat. Fat insulates the body, sheathes and protects internal organs, and provides us with a store of energy. We use it to absorb and store certain vitamins and to make some of the hormones that control body processes. It is a major component of the membranes that surround each of our cells and regulate the flow of nutrients and other substances in and out of the cell body.

Fats are composed of a small molecule called glycerol combined with one to three long molecules called fatty acids. Fats that consist of one fatty acid attached to a glycerol molecule are called monoglycerides. Diglycerides have two fatty acids attached to each glycerol, and triglycerides have three. Most of the fats in food and in the human body are triglycerides.

The fatty acids are chains of carbon atoms with oxygen and hydrogen atoms attached to them. Two oxygen atoms are attached to the carbon atom at the end of the chain. There are many carbon and hydrogen atoms, which the body can use as fuel, for each oxygen atom. This makes fats a very dense source of energy (calories). A gram of fat contains about 9 calories, while a gram of carbohydrate or protein contains only 4.

When all the spaces on a fatty acid chain that can hold a hydrogen atom are filled, it is said to be saturated. Monosaturated fatty acids are missing two hydrogen atoms. Polyunsaturated acids have unfilled spaces for four or more atoms. Polyunsaturated acids differ in the number and arrangement of the places where hydrogen atoms could fit.

Since the glycerol portion of fat molecules is the same whether the fatty acids are saturated, monosaturated, or polyunsaturated, it has become customary to simplify the nutritional information given on the labels of processed foods by labeling saturated fatty acids "saturated fat," monosaturated fatty acids "monosaturated fat," and polyunsaturated acids "polyunsaturated fat."

All the fats in food are made up of a mixture of all three fatty acid types, but the proportions vary from food to food. All kinds of fat have the same number of calories.

Currently, 15% to 20% of the calories in the American diet come from saturated fat. Saturated fats are the lipids we call "fat." They are solid at room temperature. When manufacturers want to make a solid fat out of a liquid oil, they sometimes add hydrogen to saturate additional acids—a process called hydrogenation.

About 50% of the fat in beef, lamb, and pork is saturated, as is 61% of the fat in butter and 40% of the fat in lard. Chicken contains a smaller percentage of saturated fatty acids than other meats, about 30%. The fat in dairy products is butterfat, so a high proportion of the fat in dairy products is saturated too. The butterfat in whole milk doesn't become solid and rise to the top, because homogenization breaks up the fat globules.

Fruits and vegetables are generally lower in saturated fats than are animal foods, but the most saturated fat in our diet comes from a plant: 86% of the fat in coconut oil is saturated. Coconut oil is widely used in processed foods like imitation dairy products, granola, and dry mixes.

Lipids in which monosaturated and polyunsaturated fatty acids predominate are liquid at room temperature, and we usually call them oils. Olive and peanut oil consist mostly of monosaturated fats. Many margarines and hydrogenated vegetable shortenings are also high in monosaturated fatty acids. Americans get 15% to 20% of their calories from monosaturated fats.

From 5% to 7% of the calories in the American diet come from polyunsaturated fats. Polyunsaturated fatty acids are found in the highest proportions in vegetable oils. Safflower oil is about 74% polyunsaturated, sunflower oil about 64%, corn oil about 58%, soybean and cottonseed mixtures about 40%. The fat of some fish also contains a high proportion of polyunsaturated fatty acids, and these are different in structure from the polyunsaturated fatty acids found in vegetable oils.

Because fat is such a concentrated source of energy, cutting down on fat is the best way to lose weight. However, moderate-fat diets are safer than very low-fat diets. Though the body can make many fats from sugar, starch, and protein, it cannot make three polyunsaturated fatty acids that are needed to maintain skin health and regulate growth. Very small quantities of dietary fat are sufficient to supply these essential fatty acids. Larger quantities are needed to help the body absorb the fat-soluble vitamins A, D, E, and K.

Moderate-fat diets are also easier to stick to. Fat is digested slowly, so people feel fuller after a meal that contains some fat. And fat really does make food taste better: many of the chemicals that give food its flavor and smell are easily absorbed in fat.

Cholesterol

Cholesterol is an odorless, tasteless, powdery, fatlike substance essential to animal functioning. There is no cholesterol in plants, but it is found in all animal cells, including our own, and consequently in all animal foods. Cholesterol in the human body is especially concentrated in the brain, liver, kidneys, and adrenal glands. It is an important component of the fatty sheaths surrounding nerve fibers and plays a role in the synthesis of several vital substances including sex hormones and bile salts.

Most of the cholesterol in our blood—experts' estimates vary between 70% and 80%—is manufactured by the liver. The remainder comes from dietary sources. Since the body can make its own cholesterol, we don't need to get any from food at all.

Because animal foods contain cholesterol, and animal products generally contain higher levels of saturated fat than vegetable products, cholesterol and saturated fat are often found in the same foods. They are two different kinds of substances, however, and foods may contain high levels of one and not the other. Coconut oil is high in saturated fat, for example, but is a plant product and so contains no cholesterol. Chicken fat is less saturated than beef and pork fat but contains about as much cholesterol. Both the lean part of meat, composed of muscle tissue, and the fatty part contain cholesterol; a lean cut has less saturated fat but about the same amount of cholesterol as a cut of the same weight marbled with fat. Egg yolks and organ meats are relatively low in saturated fat but high in cholesterol. Shrimp and some other seafoods are low in both total and saturated fat but high in cholesterol.

Fat and Cholesterol in the Body

Our blood, the fluids that bathe our cells, and the fluid inside our cells are all mostly water. As anyone knows who has seen an oil slick or made oil and vinegar dressing, water and oil don't mix. To make triglycerides soluble in the blood so that they can be carried to the cells, the digestive system breaks the fats into tiny drops and encases them in a shell of protein, cholesterol, and phospholipids (fatlike substances that emulsify or divide up fat). These little lipid-carrying balls are called lipoproteins. Different proteins on the shell determine where in the body cholesterol and fat will be dropped off or picked up.

Particles called chylomicrons and very low–density lipoproteins (VLDLs) carry triglycerides from the digestive tract to the liver. Chylomicrons are about 4% cholesterol; VLDLs are about 19% cholesterol. Before entering the bloodstream, VLDLs convert to low-density lipoproteins (LDLs), which are about 45% cholesterol. LDLs carry both fat and cholesterol to cells throughout the body. The cells remove the fat and cholesterol they need, converting LDLs to high-density lipoproteins (HDLs), which contain relatively little cholesterol. It is thought that HDLs pick up excess cholesterol from the body and take it back to the liver to be cleared out of the system.

The level of cholesterol in the blood is measured in milligrams (a unit of weight) per deciliter (a unit of liquid volume). There are 28,350 milligrams in an ounce. A deciliter is about a tenth of a quart. Doctors also measure the level of LDLs, HDLs, and triglycerides in the blood.

Coronary Heart Disease and Blood Cholesterol

Heart muscle, like all tissues, suffocates and dies if the blood does not supply it with oxygen. Fresh, oxygen-rich blood is carried to the heart in the coronary arteries. Atherosclerosis is a disease of the arteries in which deposits composed of cholesterol, fat, and protein accumulate on the artery walls, making them stiffer and narrower.

Heart attacks occur when a small clot or lesion or muscle spasm blocks a coronary artery, cutting off the blood supply to a piece of heart muscle. Surgeons observed years ago that the arteries cut off in heart attacks were often arteries that had already been narrowed by atherosclerosis. Researchers began studying atherosclerosis to see whether the deposits on artery walls were related to cholesterol in the blood. They compared populations of different countries and different populations within the same country and found that groups with higher levels of blood cholesterol do have more fatty deposits on their artery walls and a higher incidence of coronary heart disease (CHD). Researchers also conducted prospective studies, following a group of initially healthy people for a long period of time to see who got sick from what. They found that high blood cholesterol levels were predictive of CHD later in life. They concluded that elevated blood cholesterol is indeed a risk factor for CHD. The risk of CHD does not rise equally with every rise in blood cholesterol. There seems to be a threshold in the area of 240 milligrams per deciliter. Below that level the risk of heart disease goes up relatively modestly with each rise in blood cholesterol. As blood cholesterol levels move above 240 milligrams per deciliter, however, the risk of CHD increases dramatically.

High levels of blood cholesterol are only one of many risk factors for heart attacks. About half the risk for heart disease comes from unknown factors or factors that can't be changed, including genetic inheritance, sex, and age. Along with elevated blood cholesterol levels, cigarette smoking and high blood pressure are the main controllable factors. The various factors interact. Elevated blood cholesterol levels increase the risk of heart attack only slightly in nonsmokers with low to normal blood pressure but significantly increase the risk of heart attacks in hypertensive smokers. The degree of risk associated with elevated cholesterol levels is also influenced by age and sex. A high blood cholesterol level is a better predictor of heart attacks in middle-aged men than in men over 60. Women have not been studied as much as men.

Even when total blood cholesterol levels are somewhat elevated, a person's risk of CHD may be low if a comparatively large percentage of the total blood cholesterol is carried by protective HDL particles. Doctors generally use the total blood cholesterol level to screen patients, then measure LDL and HDL levels of those whose total cholesterol level is high.

A risk factor for a disease is not the same thing as cause of the disease. A risk factor is simply a trait or habit that occurs more frequently among people who have a disease than among people who do not. Not everyone who has one or even several risk factors for a disease will get the disease and some people will get it who have no known risk factors.

The studies that showed that high levels of blood cholesterol are associated with an increased risk of heart attack did not prove that lowering blood cholesterol would reduce the risk. Elevated blood cholesterol could be a symptom of some underlying causal condition and not a causal factor itself. To find out if lowering blood cholesterol could prevent heart attacks, researchers conducted a number of intervention studies. When a combination of drugs and diet was used to reduce cholesterol levels in men with high levels to begin with, they had fewer heart attacks than similar untreated groups. A study completed in 1987 showed that a combination of cholesterol-lowering drugs and diet actually shrank fatty deposits on implanted or natural arteries in some men who had undergone bypass surgery. Reducing blood cholesterol, researchers concluded, can indeed reduce the risk of heart disease.

Blood Cholesterol Levels and Diet

The cholesterol-lowering intervention studies all used drugs as well as diet to lower blood cholesterol, but diet alone has been shown to influence blood cholesterol levels. Though most of the cholesterol in the blood is produced in the liver, not taken from food, diet affects how the liver processes lipids. People in countries where the diet is high in fat, saturated fat, and cholesterol have higher blood cholesterol levels than the inhabitants of countries whose diet is lower in fat, saturated fat, and cholesterol. What's more, when people migrate from one country to another and adopt the eating habits of their new community, their blood cholesterol and CHD rates change accordingly.

The relationship between diet and blood cholesterol that holds true for large populations as a whole, however, shows considerable variation from individual to individual. Blood cholesterol levels are partly a matter of heredity. Some people's bodies seem to regulate cholesterol metabolism very well; they can eat a high-fat, high-cholesterol diet and still maintain healthy cholesterol levels. Others would have a high blood cholesterol level whatever their diet; they need to take drugs to bring it down. Most people's blood cholesterol levels, however, respond to changes in diet to a greater or lesser degree.

It is fat intake, not cholesterol intake, that has the strongest and most consistent effect on blood cholesterol levels. The liver appears to synthesize more cholesterol when fat supplies over 35% of the calories in the diet. The kind of fat consumed is also important. Saturated fat consumption appears to increase the production of VLDLs and LDLs, while consumption of polyunsaturated fat appears to reduce it. The effect of saturated fat is stronger: saturated fats raise blood cholesterol twice as much as polyunsaturated fats lower it. Monosaturated fats appear to have no effect on blood cholesterol levels. (A few studies suggested that monosaturated fats might have some cholesterol-lowering effects, but the results were not confirmed.)

There is more variation in people's response to dietary cholesterol than to dietary fat. When dietary intake of cholesterol is high, blood cholesterol levels rise more in some people than in others.

In 1984 the National Heart, Lung, and Blood Institute of the National Institutes of Health, in cooperation with twenty-three major medical and health organizations, released dietary recommendations based on a review of all the studies of blood cholesterol. All Americans over the age of 2 were advised to reduce total intake of fat to 30% of total calories, reduce saturated fat intake to less than 10% of total calories, increase polyunsaturated fat intake but to no more than 10% of total calories, limit daily cholesterol intake to a maximum of 300 milligrams, reduce total calories as necessary to maintain ideal body weight, and of course eat a nutritionally balanced diet. In addition, the panel urged everyone to have their cholesterol levels measured. To doctors they recommended considering adults with cholesterol levels of 240 or more as at high risk and treating them with a strict diet and if necessary with drugs; adults with blood cholesterol levels between 200 and 239 on repeated measurements should be considered borderline high, and if they have two additional risk factors (being male, smoking, a family history of CHD, high blood pressure, low levels of HDLs, severe obesity, or a history of stroke), they should be treated as high-risk patients. The revised dietary guidelines issued by the American Heart Association in 1988 made similar recommendations.

Both the National Institutes of Health Consensus Panel and the American Heart Association recommend that polyunsaturated fat constitute no more than 10% of total calories, because there is evidence that high levels of polyunsaturated fat may increase the risk for gallstones and certain cancers and may alter cell membranes. Moreover, while there are several countries where people habitually and safely consume high levels of monosaturated fats, there are no populations that consume high levels of polyunsaturated fats as part of their normal diet, so the long-term consequences of high intake are not known.

Some research suggests that consumption of certain polyunsaturated fats found in fish can lower the risk of heart disease. However, most researchers feel that the efficacy and safety of high intakes of fish oils need to be studied further before dietary recommendations are justified.

Though the consensus behind the NIH and AHA recommendations is very broad, it is not universal: a number of doctors have criticized them. These doctors generally agree that people with blood cholesterol levels above 240 (about a quarter of the adult population) should, under a doctor's supervision, lower them. But they do not feel that the evidence suggests a strong enough relationship between diet and CHD among the remainder of the population to warrant recommending a major change in the American diet as a whole, which might entail a reduction in the safety margin of nutrient consumption. They are also concerned that the emphasis on blood cholesterol levels is drawing attention away from smoking and high blood pressure. Stopping smoking and lowering blood pressure, unlike lowering blood cholesterol, have been shown not just to reduce the incidence of heart attacks, but also to extend overall life expectancy.

A larger group of critics endorses the NIH guidelines for adults but seriously questions whether they should be applied to children and adolescents, who may need more fat than adults and who need more of the nutrients contained in foods like meat and dairy products that are high in saturated fat and cholesterol.

Fat, Cholesterol, and Cancer

The relationship between dietary fat and cancer hasn't been examined as extensively as the relationships between diet, blood cholesterol, and CHD. However, there is evidence of an association between high fat intakes and certain cancers, particularly colon, prostate, and breast cancers. Polyunsaturated fats appear to promote tumor growth more than similar levels of saturated fats.

Several studies have found that very low levels of blood cholesterol are associated with a higher incidence of cancer, particularly colon cancer, and a higher overall death rate. Other studies have failed to confirm this association. More research needs to be done to determine if there is any relationship between blood cholesterol and cancer.

At present, the Committee on Diet, Nutrition, and Cancer of the National Academy of Science recommends that consumption of total fat be reduced to 30% of total calories and that the reduction be achieved by reducing intakes of both saturated and polyunsaturated fat. The calories previously supplied by these fats should be made up by increasing consumption of fruit, vegetables, and whole grain cereals and by increasing the proportion of monosaturated fat in the diet.

How to Use This Book

Food Values: Cholesterol and Fats provides the number of grams of fat and saturated fatty acids, the number of milligrams of cholesterol, and the total number of calories in thousands of foods.

The foods are divided into forty-eight categories covering all the things we eat and drink. As you flip through the pages of this book you'll quickly see where various foods are located. If you can't find a food in the category where you think it belongs, check the head note at the beginning of the category or refer to the table of contents. When products could be classified in more than one category, we have tried to include a "see also" reference.

Each category begins with an alphabetical listing of generic food items, with fresh products listed before processed foods; for instance, you'll find fresh peaches before canned peaches. Following the generic foods are all brand-name products alphabetized by the name that is most easily recognized, either the name of the manufacturing company, of the product line, or of the product itself. For instance, Campbell's soups are listed under Campbell, the company name, while Ortega sauces are listed under Ortega, the product line name, rather than under the manufacturer, Nabisco, and Kit Kat candy bar is listed under Kit Kat, because it is better known by its product name than by the fact that it is a Hershey product. Under each brand name, specific products are generally listed alphabetically; Aunt Jemima French toast, for example, precedes Aunt Jemima pancakes. We found, however, as most alphabetizers do, that some items could be listed in more than one way; we had to make choices. Fleischmann's diet margarine follows Fleischmann's regular margarine, for instance, and split peas are under *s* not *p*. If you don't find a food under the first letter of the first word of its name, try looking for it under the first letter of another word in the name. The cross-references should help here too.

Be sure to look for foods in the form in which you eat them: the way foods are prepared changes their nutrient values. A soup prepared with whole milk, for example, contains more fat, saturated fat, cholesterol, and calories than the same soup prepared with water.

We've used the portion sizes that Americans use—cups, ounces, or serving units—and when available, we've used two kinds of measures; for example, "3 cookies = 1 oz." Serving units are the easiest portions to measure: it's easier to count cookies than to weigh them. However, you can only compare serving units of the same weight. If a Brand X chocolate chip cookie weighs 1 ounce, and a Brand Y chocolate chip cookie weighs ¼ ounce, the Brand X cookie will contain more fat and cholesterol simply because it is bigger. But the Brand X chocolate chip cookie might actually contain less fat and cholesterol per unit of weight. To compare the two products you would have to multiply the values for the Brand Y cookie by 4 to find out how much fat and cholesterol it contained per ounce. When two similar products of different sizes weigh more than an ounce, divide the values for each product by the number of ounces it contains, and then compare the values per ounce for each item.

Please note the difference between weight measures and volume measures. Measuring cups measure fluid ounces. An ounce of water by weight fills a measuring cup to the 1-ounce line. But volume and weight are very different kinds of measures for solid foods. An ounce of unpopped popcorn, which is dense, wouldn't fill a measuring cup, for example, but an ounce of popped popcorn, which is airy, would fill more than one. In this book, portions for solid food given in ounces refer to weight. Fluid ounces (fl oz), cups (c), teaspoons (t), and tablespoons (T) refer to volume measurements. Since we don't ordinarily weigh our food, we've given volume and weight measurements when both are available and useful. For example, we've indicated how much of a measuring cup would be filled by an ounce of a given cold cereal when this information was available.

All the values given here are approximations. No two apples, chicken breasts, or rolls are exactly alike. Data represent averages for several samples.

Figures provided by different sources may not be exactly comparable. The U.S. Department of Agriculture (USDA) and various manufacturers may use different analytical procedures to analyze nutrient content and may round off the data in different ways. In the USDA *Composition of Food* series, our source of information about generic and fresh food, values are given to hundredths or thousandths. We rounded off the figures to the nearest whole unit. For example, we list 32.4 grams of fat as 32 grams and 32½ grams as 33 grams. When an item contained less than ½ calorie, less than ½ gram of fat, less than ½ gram of saturated fat, or less than ½ milligram of cholesterol, we listed the value as a "trace" (tr) (1 gram equals .035 ounce; 1 milligram is one-thousandth of a gram).

Many manufacturers use a simpler rounding-off system for calories, approved by the Food and Drug Administration, which regulates food labels. Calories between 0 and 20 may be given in increments of 2; between 20 and 50 in increments of 5; and above 50 in increments of 5 or 10. This means that there's no point in counting single calories when comparing products; a product listed as containing 197 calories, another listed as containing 195 calories, and a third listed as containing 200 calories may actually contain the same amount of food energy. For most practical purposes, these small differences don't matter. If you need about 2,000 calories a day, it doesn't matter if you get 2,005 one day and 1,991 the next.

This book contains the best and most complete information now available. When we could not get figures for the saturated fatty acid or cholesterol content, we put a question mark in the appropriate column. Some of this data should be available in the future. Many of the manufacturers who have not analyzed the fatty acid and cholesterol content of their products in the past intend to begin doing so now to help their customers respond to the recently issued dietary recommendations. Food manufacturers can also be expected to develop new products, change recipes, and change product sizes, so that some of the data here may quickly become outdated.

Calculating the Amount of Fat and Cholesterol in Your Diet

To get an idea of how many grams of fat and saturated fat and how many milligrams of cholesterol are in your present diet, keep a complete record of everything you eat and drink for three days, preferably including one weekend day. Right after you finish a meal or snack or cup of coffee, write down what you ate, how it was prepared, and the portion by volume (cups, tablespoons), weight (ounces, pounds), or units (one medium apple, one English muffin), or all three if you can. To get a feeling for different food sizes, measure your food when you are at home. For example, instead of just pouring milk from the carton over your cereal, pour it into a measuring cup first to see how much you use. Use tablespoons to measure the milk you pour into your tea or coffee. Look at the measurements on the side of the bar of butter or margarine and see how much you cut off when you butter your toast (a teaspoon? ½ teaspoon?). You may find that the portion sizes used in the book are smaller than the ones you use. For example, for many American adults, a typical main course portion of spaghetti is 2 cups, not the 1 cup listed as a portion here.

At the end of the three days, look up the grams of fat and saturated fat, milligrams of cholesterol, and calorie values for all the foods you have eaten. Add the figures together to get total grams of fat and saturated fat, total milligrams of cholesterol, and total calories. Divide by three to get your average daily intake.

Since saturated fat and cholesterol values are not available for many foods, particularly brand-name foods, you may have to estimate these nutrients. You can get some idea of the saturated fatty acid and cholesterol content of prepared processed foods by looking at the ingredient list on the label. By law, the ingredients are listed on the label in order of weight. If a fat or oil is at the beginning of the list, the product is probably high in fat.

The list will also tell you what kind of fat or fats the product contains. You can look these fats up in the "Fats, Oils, & Shortenings" or "Butter & Margarine Spreads" sections of this book to see whether they are high in saturated fatty acids. For example, if you look up hydrogenated soybean-cottonseed oil blends, you'll find that one cup consists of 218 grams of fat, of which 39 grams are saturated. That means these blends are about 18% saturated fat:

$$\frac{39 \text{ grams of saturated fat}}{218 \text{ grams of total fat}} = .18$$

If this book or the product label gives the number of grams of total fat in a product and you know from the ingredient list what kind of fat it contains, you can estimate the number of grams of saturated fat in the food. For example, if the label says that one serving of the product contains 14 grams of fat, and the only fat listed as an ingredient is hydrogenated soybean-cottonseed oil (18% saturated), then the serving contains about 14 times 18% (.18) grams of saturated fat, or 2½ grams. Products that contain only trace amounts of total fat can of course contain only trace amounts of saturated fat. Products that contain no ingredients of animal origin contain no cholesterol.

Following the National Institutes of Health Guidelines

The National Institutes of Health and the American Heart Association recommend that everyone limit cholesterol intake to a maximum of 300 milligrams a day. To bring your diet into conformity with this recommendation, all you have to do is calculate your average daily intake of cholesterol, and then, if it is over 300 milligrams, start eliminating or reducing your portions of high-cholesterol foods. The recommendations about fat and saturated fat are a little harder to follow, since they are given in terms of percentage of total calories: we are advised to reduce fat consumption to 30% of total calories, saturated fat consumption to 10% of total calories.

To find the number of calories supplied by fat in a given food, multiply the number of grams of fat in the food by 9, the number of calories in a gram of fat. To find the percentage of calories supplied by fat, divide the number of calories obtained from fat by the total number of calories. For example, a cup of baked custard contains 15 grams of fat. That means 9 times 15, or 135, calories are supplied by fat. The total number of calories in a cup of custard is 305. The percentage of those calories supplied by fat is $^{135}/_{305}$, or 44%.

You can use the same procedure to find the percentage of calories supplied by saturated fat: multiply grams of saturated fat by 9 and divide by total calories. To use the same example, the cup of custard contains about 7 grams of saturated fat, which provide 7 times 9, or 63, calories, so $^{63}/_{305}$ of the total calories, or 20%, come from saturated fat.

To calculate the percentage of calories supplied by fat or saturated fat in a given meal, add together all the grams of fat (or saturated fat) in each of the foods, multiply by 9, and divide by the total number of calories in the meal.

You will probably find it's easiest to think of your fat intake in terms of whole days, not meals or individual foods. That way you can allow for the occasional gourmet ice cream cone by reducing the fat content of your other meals that day.

The percentage of calories provided by fat in your present diet is equal to your average daily intake of fat times 9, divided by your average daily intake of calories:

$$\frac{\text{average daily intake of fat} \times 9}{\text{average daily intake of calories}} = \% \text{ calories from fat}$$

For saturated fat, the formula is:

$$\frac{\text{average daily intake of saturated fat} \times 9}{\text{average daily intake of calories}} = \% \text{ calories from saturated fat}$$

For example, if you eat 85 grams of fat on the average, you get an average of 85 times 9 calories from fat every day—765. If your average total caloric intake is 2,000 calories a day, you are getting about $^{765}/_{2,000}$, or 38%, of your calories

from fat. To follow the NIH and AHA recommendations, you
will have to reduce your fat intake to about 30% of total
calories. For example, if your daily caloric intake is 2,000
calories, 30% of that intake is 2,000 times .3, or 600 calories. To find out how many grams of fat provide a given
number of calories, divide the given number of calories by
9. For example, if you want to get 600 calories from fat, you
can eat $\frac{600}{9}$ or 66⅔ grams of fat.

You can do this calculation in one step:

average daily caloric intake × .033 = grams of fat
needed to supply
30% of daily calo-
ric intake

No more than one-third of your total fat intake should come
from saturated fat:

$$\frac{\text{allowable grams of fat}}{3} = \frac{\text{allowable grams of saturated fat}}{\text{(10\% of daily caloric intake)}}$$

or:

average daily caloric intake × .011 = grams of fat
needed to supply
10% of daily calo-
ric intake

For example, if 66⅔ grams of fat will provide 30% of your
total daily caloric intake, you should limit your intake of
saturated fats to 22.2 grams of saturated fat.

The following chart may be helpful.

Daily Calories	Grams of Fat = 30% of Daily Calories	Grams of Saturated Fat = 10% of Daily Calories
1,500	50	16–17
1,800	60	20
2,000	67	22–23
2,250	75	25
2,500	83	27–28
2,700	90	30
3,000	100	33–34

If you want to calculate the percentage of calories supplied by fat in a product by using information on the label, once again, multiply the number of grams of total fat by 9 and divide by the total calories. The percentage of calories supplied by fat will be much higher than the percentage of weight that is fat, because fat has more than twice as many calories per unit of weight than either protein or carbohydrate and also because water, a major ingredient by weight of many foods, contributes no calories at all. For example, when milk is labeled 3.3% fat, that means that 3.3% of the weight of the milk is fat, or to put it another way, that 100 grams of this milk contain 3.3 grams of fat. Those 3.3 grams provide 3.3 times 9 or 29.7 calories. The total number of calories in 100 grams of milk is 61, so $^{29.7}/_{61}$, or 49%, of those calories come from fat. This is important to note: some products that advertise themselves as "less than 5% fat" or "less than 2% fat" are actually comparatively fatty.

These formulas aren't precise. The amount of energy the body gets from fat, carbohydrate, and protein varies slightly from food to food. But the method is accurate enough for good meal planning and is the method used by many nutritionists working at schools and other institutions.

Nutrition isn't a definitive science; recommendations about the most healthful diet are made on the basis of the evidence we have now. That evidence is still incomplete—which is why, when it comes to diet, doctors often disagree. The one recommendation about which there is a consensus is that the most healthful diet is a moderate, balanced one, which includes a variety of foods—and tastes good enough so that people will stick to it. We hope this book will help you find tasty ways to reduce the amount of fat and cholesterol in your diet.

Sources

1. *Food Values of Portions Commonly Used, 14th Edition*, Jean A. T. Pennington and Helen Nichols Church, Harper & Row, 1985.
2. *Nutritive Value of Foods*, U.S. Department of Agriculture, Nutrition Information Service, Home and Garden Bulletin #72, revised 1981.
3. *Composition of Food Series*, U.S. Department of Agriculture, Science and Education Administration:

   8-1 *Dairy and Egg Products*, revised November 1976.

   8-3 *Baby Foods*, revised December 1978.

   8-4 *Fats and Oils*, revised June 1979.

   8-5 *Poultry Products*, revised August 1979.

   8-6 *Soups, Sauces and Gravies*, revised February 1980.

   8-7 *Sausages and Luncheon Meats*, revised September 1980.

   8-8 *Breakfast Cereals*, revised July 1982.

   8-9 *Fruits and Fruit Juices*, revised August 1982.

   8-10 *Pork Products*, revised August 1983.

   8-11 *Vegetables and Vegetable Products*, revised August 1984.

   8-12 *Nut and Seed Products*, revised September 1984.

   8-13 *Beef Products*, revised August 1986.

   8-14 *Beverages*, revised May 1986.

   8-15 *Finfish and Shellfish Products*, revised September 1987.

   8-16 *Legumes and Legume Products*, revised December 1986.

Information about brand-name products was supplied by the food processing companies themselves or taken from the above sources.

Abbreviations

c	=	cup
cal	=	calories
chol	=	cholesterol
diam	=	diameter
g	=	grams
lb	=	pounds
mg	=	milligrams
oz	=	ounces
pkg	=	package
pkt	=	packet
sat fat	=	saturated fat
T	=	tablespoon
t	=	teaspoon
tr	=	trace
w/	=	with
w/out	=	without
?	=	not available, or not known at this time
<	=	less than
≤	=	less than or equal to

	Portion	Chol (mg)	Total Fat (g)	Satur'd Fat (g)	Total Calor

▢ ALCOHOLIC BEVERAGES
See BEVERAGES

▢ BABY FOOD *See* INFANT & TODDLER FOODS

▢ BAKING INGREDIENTS

	Portion	Chol (mg)	Total Fat (g)	Satur'd Fat (g)	Total Calor
baking powder, all types	1 t	0	0	0	5
baking soda	1 t	0	0	0	0
candied fruit					
apricot	1 medium	0	tr	?	101
cherry	3 large	0	tr	?	51
maraschino cherry	2 medium	0	tr	?	19
citron	1 oz	0	tr	?	89
fig	1 piece	0	tr	?	90
ginger root	1 oz	0	tr	?	95
peel of grapefruit/lemon/ orange	1 oz	0	tr	?	89
pear	1 oz	0	tr	?	85
pineapple	1 slice	0	tr	?	120
cornmeal *See* FLOURS & CORNMEALS					
cornstarch *See* FLOURS & CORNMEALS					
flour *See* FLOURS & CORNMEALS					
pastry puff dough	1 oz	?	10	?	129
patty shell	2½ oz	?	19	?	240
piecrust					
crumb	5.8 oz	?	64	?	866
from mix, w/vegetable shortening	for 2-crust 9″ pie	0	93	23	1,485
from sticks	⅙ double crust = 2 oz	?	18	?	290
frozen	1⁄16 crust = 1 oz	5	8	?	130
graham cracker	4.8 oz	?	10	?	159
homemade, w/vegetable shortening	for 9″ pie	0	60	15	900
yeast					
baker's, dry, active	1 pkg	0	tr	tr	20
brewer's, dry	1 T	0	tr	tr	25
torula	1 T	0	tr	tr	28

	Portion	Chol (mg)	Total Fat (g)	Satur'd Fat (g)	Total Calor
■ BRAND NAME					
Baker's					
COCONUT					
Angel Flake, bag	⅓ c	0	8	?	120
CHOCOLATE					
German's sweet chocolate	1 oz	0	10	?	140
semisweet chocolate	1 oz	0	9	?	140
semisweet chocolate–flavored chips	¼ c	0	9	?	190
semisweet real chocolate chips	¼ c	0	12	?	200
unsweetened chocolate	1 oz	0	15	?	140
Davis					
baking powder	1 t	?	0	?	8
Hershey					
milk chocolate chips	1 oz	?	8	?	150
semisweet chocolate chips, regular & miniature	¼ c or 1½ oz	?	12	?	220
unsweetened baking chocolate	1 oz	4	16	10	190
Nabisco					
graham cracker crumbs	2 T	?	1	?	60
Reese's					
peanut butter–flavored chips	¼ c or 1½ oz	3	13	11	230
Sunshine					
graham cracker crumbs	1 c	0	14	?	550

▢ BAKING MIXES

	Portion	Chol (mg)	Total Fat (g)	Satur'd Fat (g)	Total Calor
all-purpose biscuit/pancake mix	½ c	?	8	?	240

cakes & pastries, prepared from mix *See* DESSERTS: CAKES, PASTRIES, & PIES
pancakes, prepared from mix *See* BREAKFAST FOODS, PREPARED
pie fillings, prepared from mix *See* DESSERTS: CUSTARDS, GELATINS, PUDDINGS, & PIE FILLINGS
waffles, prepared from mix *See* BREAKFAST FOODS, PREPARED

	Portion	Chol (mg)	Total Fat (g)	Satur'd Fat (g)	Total Calor
■ BRAND NAME					
Arrowhead Mills					
biscuit mix	2 oz	tr	1	?	100
bran muffin mix	2 muffins	tr	7	?	270

	Portion	Chol (mg)	Total Fat (g)	Satur'd Fat (g)	Total Calor
corn bread mix	1 oz	tr	1	?	100
Aunt Jemima					
Easy Mix coffee cake	1.3 oz	?	4	?	162
Easy Mix corn bread	1.7 oz	?	6	?	205
Dromedary					
corn bread, prepared	2″×2″ piece	?	3	?	130
corn muffin, prepared	1 muffin	?	4	?	120
gingerbread, prepared	2″×2″ piece	?	2	?	100
pound cake, prepared	½″ slice	?	6	?	150
Fearn					
BAKING MIXES					
brown rice	½ c	0	3	tr	215
rice	½ c	0	1	tr	260
whole-wheat	½ c	1	2	tr	210
BREAD & MUFFIN MIXES					
bran muffin	1½ oz	tr	1	tr	110
corn bread	⅓ c dry	1	2	tr	160
CAKE MIXES					
banana	⅓ c dry	1	2	tr	130
carob	⅓ c dry	tr	2	tr	120
carrot	⅓ c dry	tr	2	tr	140
spice	⅓ c dry	1	3	1	140
Flako					
corn muffin mix	1 oz	?	2	?	116
pie crust mix	1.7 oz	?	14	?	244
popover mix	1 oz	?	1	?	102
Jell-O					
cheesecake, prepared w/ whole milk	⅛ of 8″ cake	30	13	?	280
chocolate mousse pie, prepared w/whole milk	⅛ pie	30	15	?	250
coconut cream pie, prepared w/whole milk	⅛ pie	30	17	?	260
Pillsbury					
All Ready pie crust	⅛ of 2-crust pie	?	15	?	240
Royal					
chocolate mint pie mix	⅛ pie	?	15	?	260
chocolate mousse pie mix	⅛ pie	?	12	?	230
lemon meringue pie mix	⅛ pie	?	11	?	310
lite cheese cake mix	⅛ pie	?	10	?	210
Real cheese cake mix	⅛ pie	?	9	?	280

	Portion	Chol (mg)	Total Fat (g)	Satur'd Fat (g)	Total Calor

❑ BEANS *See* LEGUMES & LEGUME PRODUCTS

❑ BEEF, FRESH & CURED
See also PROCESSED MEAT & POULTRY PRODUCTS

NOTE: "1 lb raw" refers to the edible portion of meat yielded when 1 pound of the raw product is cooked.

Beef, Fresh

BRISKET
Lean & Fat

	Portion	Chol (mg)	Total Fat (g)	Satur'd Fat (g)	Total Calor
whole, all grades, braised	3 oz cooked	79	28	11	332
	1 lb raw	301	104	42	1,258
flat half, all grades, braised	3 oz cooked	78	30	12	347
	1 lb raw	296	112	46	1,311
point half, all grades, braised	3 oz cooked	81	25	10	311
	1 lb raw	304	93	38	1,172

Lean Only

	Portion	Chol (mg)	Total Fat (g)	Satur'd Fat (g)	Total Calor
whole, all grades, braised	3 oz cooked	79	11	4	205
	1 lb raw	197	27	10	513
flat half, all grades, braised	3 oz cooked	77	13	5	223
	1 lb raw	190	33	13	549
point half, all grades, braised	3 oz cooked	81	7	3	181
	1 lb raw	206	19	7	461

CHUCK, ARM ROAST
Lean & Fat

	Portion	Chol (mg)	Total Fat (g)	Satur'd Fat (g)	Total Calor
all grades, braised	3 oz cooked	84	22	9	297
	1 lb raw	273	71	29	962
choice, braised	3 oz cooked	84	23	9	301
	1 lb raw	274	73	30	982
good, braised	3 oz cooked	84	21	9	287
	1 lb raw	263	65	27	894
prime, braised	3 oz cooked	84	26	11	332
	1 lb raw	274	86	35	1,082

	Portion	Chol (mg)	Total Fat (g)	Satur'd Fat (g)	Total Calor
Lean Only					
all grades, braised	3 oz cooked	85	8	3	196
	1 lb raw	203	20	8	467
choice, braised	3 oz cooked	85	7	3	199
	1 lb raw	203	18	8	473
good, braised	3 oz cooked	85	8	3	189
	1 lb raw	199	18	7	439
prime, braised	3 oz cooked	85	11	4	222
	1 lb raw	192	26	10	499
CHUCK, BLADE ROAST					
Lean & Fat					
all grades, braised	3 oz cooked	87	26	11	325
	1 lb raw	258	76	32	961
choice, braised	3 oz cooked	87	26	11	330
	1 lb raw	260	78	33	982
good, braised	3 oz cooked	88	24	10	311
	1 lb raw	248	68	29	882
prime, braised	3 oz cooked	87	29	12	354
	1 lb raw	254	84	35	1,029
Lean Only					
all grades, braised	3 oz cooked	90	13	5	230
	1 lb raw	192	28	11	492
choice, braised	3 oz cooked	90	13	5	234
	1 lb raw	193	29	12	503
good, braised	3 oz cooked	90	12	5	218
	1 lb raw	188	24	10	456
prime, braised	3 oz cooked	90	17	7	270
	1 lb raw	189	37	15	569
FLANK					
Lean & Fat					
choice braised	3 oz cooked	61	13	6	218
	1 lb raw	193	41	18	689

	Portion	Chol (mg)	Total Fat (g)	Satur'd Fat (g)	Total Calor
choice *(cont.)*					
broiled	3 oz cooked	60	14	6	216
	1 lb raw	241	55	24	863
Lean Only					
choice					
braised	3 oz cooked	60	12	5	208
	1 lb raw	185	36	15	635
broiled	3 oz cooked	60	13	5	207
	1 lb raw	233	50	21	808
GROUND BEEF					
Extra Lean					
baked					
medium	3 oz cooked	70	14	5	213
	1 lb raw	283	56	22	863
well done	3 oz cooked	91	14	5	232
	1 lb raw	286	43	17	733
broiled					
medium	3 oz cooked	71	14	5	217
	1 lb raw	281	55	22	859
well done	3 oz cooked	84	13	5	225
	1 lb raw	277	44	17	744
pan-fried					
medium	3 oz cooked	69	14	5	216
	1 lb raw	274	56	22	866
well done	3 oz cooked	79	14	5	224
	1 lb raw	275	47	18	777
Lean					
baked					
medium	3 oz cooked	66	16	6	227
	1 lb raw	262	62	24	899
well done	3 oz cooked	84	16	6	248
	1 lb raw	261	48	19	768
broiled					
medium	3 oz cooked	74	16	6	231
	1 lb raw	240	59	23	876

	Portion	Chol (mg)	Total Fat (g)	Satur'd Fat (g)	Total Calor
well done	3 oz cooked	86	15	6	238
	1 lb raw	283	50	19	785
pan-fried medium	3 oz cooked	71	16	6	234
	1 lb raw	275	62	24	901
well done	3 oz cooked	81	15	6	235
	1 lb raw	273	51	20	791
Regular					
baked medium	3 oz cooked	74	18	7	244
	1 lb raw	276	67	26	913
well done	3 oz cooked	92	18	7	269
	1 lb raw	274	55	21	804
broiled medium	3 oz cooked	76	18	7	246
	1 lb raw	273	63	25	880
well done	3 oz cooked	86	17	7	248
	1 lb raw	274	53	21	793
pan-fried medium	3 oz cooked	75	19	8	260
	1 lb raw	273	69	27	941
well done	3 oz cooked	83	16	6	243
	1 lb raw	272	52	21	792
GROUND, FROZEN PATTIES					
broiled, medium	3 oz cooked	80	17	7	240
	1 lb raw	294	62	24	882
RIB, WHOLE (RIBS 6–12)					
Lean & Fat					
all grades broiled	3 oz cooked	73	25	11	308
	1 lb raw	245	86	36	1,039
roasted	3 oz cooked	72	27	11	324
	1 lb raw	233	87	37	1,042

	Portion	Chol (mg)	Total Fat (g)	Satur'd Fat (g)	Total Calor
choice					
broiled	3 oz cooked	73	26	11	313
	1 lb raw	247	88	37	1,060
roasted	3 oz cooked	72	28	12	328
	1 lb raw	234	89	38	1,062
good					
broiled	3 oz cooked	72	23	10	289
	1 lb raw	242	78	33	969
roasted	3 oz cooked	72	25	11	306
	1 lb raw	230	80	34	978
prime					
broiled	3 oz cooked	73	30	13	347
	1 lb raw	253	104	44	1,199
roasted	3 oz cooked	73	31	13	361
	1 lb raw	239	103	44	1,189
Lean Only					
all grades					
broiled	3 oz cooked	69	11	5	194
	1 lb raw	165	26	11	461
roasted	3 oz cooked	68	12	5	204
	1 lb raw	150	26	11	449
choice					
broiled	3 oz cooked	69	12	5	198
	1 lb raw	164	27	11	469
roasted	3 oz cooked	68	12	5	209
	1 lb raw	149	27	11	456
good					
broiled	3 oz cooked	69	10	4	181
	1 lb raw	169	23	10	440
roasted	3 oz cooked	68	10	4	191
	1 lb raw	153	23	10	430
prime					
broiled	3 oz cooked	69	16	7	238
	1 lb raw	164	38	16	562
roasted	3 oz cooked	68	17	7	248
	1 lb raw	148	36	15	536

	Portion	Chol (mg)	Total Fat (g)	Satur'd Fat (g)	Total Calor
RIB, EYE, SMALL END (RIBS 10–12)					
Lean & Fat					
choice, broiled	3 oz cooked	70	18	7	250
	1 lb raw	271	68	29	966
Lean Only					
choice, broiled	3 oz cooked	68	10	4	191
	1 lb raw	223	32	15	623
RIB, LARGE END (RIBS 6–9)					
Lean & Fat					
all grades					
broiled	3 oz cooked	74	27	12	321
	1 lb raw	248	93	39	1,083
roasted	3 oz cooked	72	26	11	313
	1 lb raw	237	84	35	1,030
choice					
broiled	3 oz cooked	74	28	12	327
	1 lb raw	249	95	40	1,107
roasted	3 oz cooked	72	26	11	316
	1 lb raw	237	85	36	1,040
good					
broiled	3 oz cooked	73	25	11	301
	1 lb raw	246	84	36	1,009
roasted	3 oz cooked	72	24	10	304
	1 lb raw	237	81	34	1,000
prime					
broiled	3 oz cooked	74	32	14	361
	1 lb raw	259	112	48	1,267
roasted	3 oz cooked	72	29	13	346
	1 lb raw	238	97	41	1,136
Lean Only					
all grades					
broiled	3 oz cooked	70	12	5	198
	1 lb raw	160	28	12	453

	Portion	Chol (mg)	Total Fat (g)	Satur'd Fat (g)	Total Calor
all grades *(cont.)*					
roasted	3 oz cooked	68	12	5	207
	1 lb raw	161	28	12	487
choice					
broiled	3 oz cooked	70	13	5	203
	1 lb raw	160	29	12	464
roasted	3 oz cooked	68	12	7	210
	1 lb raw	161	29	16	495
good					
broiled	3 oz cooked	70	10	4	183
	1 lb raw	164	24	10	428
roasted	3 oz cooked	68	11	5	197
	1 lb raw	163	26	11	468
prime					
broiled	3 oz cooked	70	18	8	250
	1 lb raw	162	41	18	575
roasted	3 oz cooked	68	16	7	241
	1 lb raw	155	35	15	543

RIB, SMALL END (RIBS 10–12)

Lean & Fat

	Portion	Chol (mg)	Total Fat (g)	Satur'd Fat (g)	Total Calor
all grades					
broiled	3 oz cooked	71	21	9	277
	1 lb raw	244	72	31	950
roasted	3 oz cooked	72	25	11	305
	1 lb raw	231	80	34	981
choice					
broiled	3 oz cooked	71	22	9	282
	1 lb raw	244	74	31	965
roasted	3 oz cooked	72	26	11	312
	1 lb raw	231	82	35	1,002
good					
broiled	3 oz cooked	71	19	8	263
	1 lb raw	240	66	28	889
roasted	3 oz cooked	72	22	9	283
	1 lb raw	227	71	30	900

	Portion	Chol (mg)	Total Fat (g)	Satur'd Fat (g)	Total Calor
prime					
broiled	3 oz cooked	71	25	10	309
	1 lb raw	240	83	35	1,041
roasted	3 oz cooked	72	31	13	357
	1 lb raw	231	99	42	1,142
Lean Only					
all grades					
broiled	3 oz cooked	68	10	4	188
	1 lb raw	179	25	11	492
roasted	3 oz cooked	68	11	5	201
	1 lb raw	159	27	11	465
choice					
broiled	3 oz cooked	68	10	4	191
	1 lb raw	178	26	11	499
roasted	3 oz cooked	68	12	5	206
	1 lb raw	158	28	12	476
good					
broiled	3 oz cooked	68	8	4	178
	1 lb raw	182	22	9	473
roasted	3 oz cooked	68	10	4	183
	1 lb raw	162	23	10	433
prime					
broiled	3 oz cooked	68	13	6	221
	1 lb raw	173	33	14	559
roasted	3 oz cooked	68	18	8	259
	1 lb raw	151	40	17	572
RIB, SHORT					
Lean & Fat					
choice, braised	3 oz cooked	80	36	15	400
	1 lb raw	212	95	40	1,064
Lean Only					
choice, braised	3 oz cooked	79	15	7	251
	1 lb raw	114	22	10	363

	Portion	Chol (mg)	Total Fat (g)	Satur'd Fat (g)	Total Calor
ROUND, FULL CUT					
Lean & Fat					
choice, broiled	3 oz cooked	71	16	6	233
	1 lb raw	255	55	22	832
good, broiled	3 oz cooked	71	14	6	222
	1 lb raw	253	51	20	790
Lean Only					
choice, broiled	3 oz cooked	70	7	2	165
	1 lb raw	208	20	7	493
good, broiled	3 oz cooked	70	6	2	157
	1 lb raw	209	18	6	470
ROUND, BOTTOM					
Lean & Fat					
all grades, braised	3 oz cooked	81	13	5	222
	1 lb raw	266	41	16	725
choice, braised	3 oz cooked	81	13	5	224
	1 lb raw	266	42	16	734
good, braised	3 oz cooked	81	12	5	215
	1 lb raw	265	38	15	700
prime, braised	3 oz cooked	81	16	6	253
	1 lb raw	275	59	21	853
Lean Only					
all grades, braised	3 oz cooked	81	8	3	189
	1 lb raw	243	25	9	564
choice, braised	3 oz cooked	81	8	3	191
	1 lb raw	243	25	9	571
good, braised	3 oz cooked	81	7	3	182
	1 lb raw	243	22	8	543
prime, braised	3 oz cooked	81	11	4	212
	1 lb raw	239	32	11	622

	Portion	Chol (mg)	Total Fat (g)	Satur'd Fat (g)	Total Calor
ROUND, EYE OF					
Lean & Fat					
all grades, roasted	3 oz cooked	62	12	5	206
	1 lb raw	260	51	21	869
choice, roasted	3 oz cooked	62	12	5	207
	1 lb raw	259	51	21	871
good, roasted	3 oz cooked	62	12	5	201
	1 lb raw	260	49	20	851
prime, roasted	3 oz cooked	61	13	5	213
	1 lb raw	256	53	21	888
Lean Only					
all grades, roasted	3 oz cooked	59	6	2	155
	1 lb raw	219	21	8	575
choice, roasted	3 oz cooked	59	6	2	156
	1 lb raw	218	21	8	578
good, roasted	3 oz cooked	59	5	2	151
	1 lb raw	219	19	7	562
prime, roasted	3 oz cooked	59	7	3	168
	1 lb raw	220	26	10	628
ROUND, TIP					
Lean & Fat					
all grades, roasted	3 oz cooked	70	13	5	213
	1 lb raw	272	50	20	823
choice, roasted	3 oz cooked	70	13	5	216
	1 lb raw	273	52	21	837
good, roasted	3 oz cooked	70	12	5	205
	1 lb raw	268	46	18	780
prime, roasted	3 oz cooked	71	16	7	242
	1 lb raw	273	63	25	932
Lean Only					
all grades, roasted	3 oz cooked	69	6	2	162
	1 lb raw	233	22	8	546

	Portion	Chol (mg)	Total Fat (g)	Satur'd Fat (g)	Total Calor
choice, roasted	3 oz cooked	69	7	2	164
	1 lb raw	233	22	8	552
good, roasted	3 oz cooked	69	6	2	156
	1 lb raw	232	19	7	524
prime, roasted	3 oz cooked	69	9	3	181
	1 lb raw	225	28	10	593
ROUND, TOP					
Lean & Fat					
all grades, broiled	3 oz cooked	72	7	3	179
	1 lb raw	281	29	11	701
choice					
broiled	3 oz cooked	72	8	3	181
	1 lb raw	282	30	11	709
pan-fried	3 oz cooked	82	15	6	246
	1 lb raw	274	48	18	819
good, broiled	3 oz cooked	72	7	3	176
	1 lb raw	281	28	10	686
prime, broiled	3 oz cooked	72	10	4	201
	1 lb raw	281	39	14	783
Lean Only					
all grades, broiled	3 oz cooked	72	5	2	162
	1 lb raw	269	20	7	610
choice					
broiled	3 oz cooked	72	5	2	165
	1 lb raw	269	21	7	617
pan-fried	3 oz cooked	83	7	2	193
	1 lb raw	238	21	7	556
good, broiled	3 oz cooked	72	5	2	156
	1 lb raw	267	17	6	583
prime, broiled	3 oz cooked	72	8	3	183
	1 lb raw	265	28	10	678

	Portion	Chol (mg)	Total Fat (g)	Satur'd Fat (g)	Total Calor
SHANK CROSSCUTS					
Lean & Fat					
choice, simmered	3 oz cooked	67	10	4	208
	1 lb raw	165	25	10	508
Lean Only					
choice, simmered	3 oz cooked	66	5	2	171
	1 lb raw	147	12	4	380
SHORT LOIN, PORTERHOUSE STEAK					
Lean & Fat					
choice, broiled	3 oz cooked	70	18	7	254
	1 lb raw	222	57	24	803
Lean Only					
choice, broiled	3 oz cooked	68	9	4	185
	1 lb raw	178	24	10	483
SHORT LOIN, T-BONE STEAK					
Lean & Fat					
choice, broiled	3 oz cooked	71	21	9	276
	1 lb raw	229	67	28	888
Lean Only					
choice, broiled	3 oz cooked	68	9	4	182
	1 lb raw	167	22	9	447
SHORT LOIN, TENDERLOIN					
Lean & Fat					
all grades broiled	3 oz cooked	73	15	6	226
	1 raw steak, edible portion = 4 oz	99	20	8	306

	Portion	Chol (mg)	Total Fat (g)	Satur'd Fat (g)	Total Calor
all grades *(cont.)*					
roasted	3 oz cooked	74	19	8	258
	1 raw steak, edible portion = 4.2 oz	105	26	11	364
choice					
broiled	3 oz cooked	73	15	6	230
	1 raw steak, edible portion = 4.1 oz	100	21	8	314
roasted	3 oz cooked	74	19	8	262
	1 raw steak, edible portion = 4.2 oz	105	27	11	370
good					
broiled	3 oz cooked	73	13	5	216
	1 raw steak, edible portion = 4 oz	97	18	7	286
roasted	3 oz cooked	74	17	7	245
	1 raw steak, edible portion = 4.2 oz	104	24	10	343
prime					
broiled	3 oz cooked	73	20	8	270
	1 raw steak, edible portion = 4 oz	99	27	11	362

	Portion	Chol (mg)	Total Fat (g)	Satur'd Fat (g)	Total Calor
roasted	3 oz cooked	75	24	10	305
	1 raw steak, edible portion = 4.1 oz	102	33	14	416
Lean Only					
all grades					
broiled	3 oz cooked	72	8	3	174
	1 raw steak, edible portion = 3½ oz	84	9	7	204
roasted	3 oz cooked	73	10	4	186
	1 raw steak, edible portion = 3½ oz	84	11	4	215
choice					
broiled	3 oz cooked	72	8	3	176
	1 raw steak, edible portion = 3.6 oz	85	10	4	209
roasted	3 oz cooked	73	10	4	189
	1 raw steak, edible portion = 3.4 oz	83	11	4	216
good					
broiled	3 oz cooked	72	7	3	167
	1 raw steak, edible portion = 3½ oz	84	8	3	196

	Portion	Chol (mg)	Total Fat (g)	Satur'd Fat (g)	Total Calor
good *(cont.)*					
roasted	3 oz cooked	73	9	3	177
	1 raw steak, edible portion = 3½ oz	85	10	4	206
prime					
broiled	3 oz cooked	72	11	4	197
	1 raw steak, edible portion = 3.2 oz	78	11	4	214
roasted	3 oz cooked	73	13	5	217
	1 raw steak, edible portion = 3.1 oz	75	13	5	225
SHORT LOIN, TOP					
Lean & Fat					
all grades, broiled	3 oz cooked	67	16	7	238
	1 raw steak, edible portion = 8.2 oz	185	44	18	651
choice, broiled	3 oz cooked	68	17	7	243
	1 raw steak, edible portion = 8.3 oz	187	46	19	672
good, broiled	3 oz cooked	67	14	6	223
	1 raw steak, edible portion = 8.1 oz	182	39	16	603

	Portion	Chol (mg)	Total Fat (g)	Satur'd Fat (g)	Total Calor
prime, broiled	3 oz cooked	68	22	9	288
	1 raw steak, edible portion = 8.1 oz	183	59	24	774
Lean Only					
all grades, broiled	3 oz cooked	65	8	3	172
	1 raw steak, edible portion = 6.9 oz	149	17	7	395
choice, broiled	3 oz cooked	65	8	3	176
	1 raw steak, edible portion = 6.9 oz	150	18	7	406
good, broiled	3 oz cooked	65	6	3	162
	1 raw steak, edible portion = 6.9 oz	150	15	6	373
prime, broiled	3 oz cooked	65	12	5	208
	1 raw steak, edible portion = 6.3 oz	137	24	10	438
WEDGE-BONE SIRLOIN					
Lean & Fat					
all grades, broiled	3 oz cooked	77	15	6	238
	1 lb raw	255	51	21	791
choice broiled	3 oz cooked	77	16	7	240
	1 lb raw	256	52	22	804
pan-fried	3 oz cooked	84	21	9	288
	1 lb raw	265	66	27	913

	Portion	Chol (mg)	Total Fat (g)	Satur'd Fat (g)	Total Calor
good, broiled	3 oz cooked	77	15	6	232
	1 lb raw	256	49	21	777
prime, broiled	3 oz cooked	77	19	8	271
	1 lb raw	248	63	26	878
Lean Only					
all grades, broiled	3 oz cooked	76	7	3	177
	1 lb raw	214	21	9	500
choice					
broiled	3 oz cooked	76	8	3	180
	1 lb raw	215	22	9	509
pan-fried	3 oz cooked	85	9	4	202
	1 lb raw	206	23	9	492
good, broiled	3 oz cooked	76	7	3	170
	1 lb raw	215	19	8	482
prime, broiled	3 oz cooked	76	10	4	201
	1 lb raw	199	26	11	527
VARIETY MEATS					
brains					
pan-fried	3 oz cooked	1,696	13	3	167
	1 lb raw	7,003	56	13	690
simmered	3 oz cooked	1,746	11	2	136
	1 lb raw	8,030	49	11	627
heart, simmered	3 oz cooked	164	5	1	148
	1 lb raw	496	14	4	450
kidneys, simmered	3 oz cooked	329	3	1	122
	1 lb raw	762	7	2	283
liver					
braised	3 oz cooked	331	4	2	137
	1 lb raw	1,308	16	6	542
pan-fried	3 oz cooked	410	7	2	184
	1 lb raw	1,423	24	8	639
lungs, braised	3 oz cooked	236	3	1	102
	1 lb raw	840	11	3	365
suet, raw	1 oz	19	27	15	242

	Portion	Chol (mg)	Total Fat (g)	Satur'd Fat (g)	Total Calor
tongue, simmered	3 oz cooked	91	18	8	241
	1 lb raw	278	54	23	732
tripe, raw	1 oz	27	1	1	28
	4 oz	107	4	2	111

Beef, Cured

	Portion	Chol (mg)	Total Fat (g)	Satur'd Fat (g)	Total Calor
breakfast strips, cooked	3 (15 per 12 oz pkg)	40	12	5	153
	6 oz	202	58	24	764
corned beef brisket, braised	3 oz cooked	83	16	5	213
	1 lb raw	314	61	20	802

▪ BRAND NAME

Oscar Mayer

	Portion	Chol (mg)	Total Fat (g)	Satur'd Fat (g)	Total Calor
breakfast strips, cooked	1 (15 per 12 oz pkg)	13	4	2	46

▫ BEVERAGES

See also FAST FOODS; MILK, MILK SUBSTITUTES, & MILK PRODUCTS

Beverages, Alcoholic

BEER & ALE

Beer & ale contain virtually no cholesterol or fat.

COCKTAILS & MIXED DRINKS

	Portion	Chol (mg)	Total Fat (g)	Satur'd Fat (g)	Total Calor
Bloody Mary, daiquiri, gin & tonic, manhattan, martini, screwdriver, tequila sunrise, Tom Collins, whiskey sour	2–8 fl oz	0	0 or tr	0 or tr	varies
eggnog *See* Flavored Milk Beverages, *below*					
piña colada, canned	6.8 fl oz	?	17	15	525
piña colada cocktail	4½ fl oz	0	3	1	262

CORDIALS & LIQUEURS

	Portion	Chol (mg)	Total Fat (g)	Satur'd Fat (g)	Total Calor
54 proof (22.1% alcohol by weight)	1 fl oz	0	0	0	97
coffee liqueur (53 proof)	1½ fl oz	0	tr	tr	174
coffee w/cream liqueur (34 proof)	1½ fl oz	?	7	5	154

	Portion	Chol (mg)	Total Fat (g)	Satur'd Fat (g)	Total Calor
crème de menthe liqueur (72 proof)	1½ fl oz	0	tr	tr	186
DISTILLED SPIRITS					
all (gin, rum, vodka, whiskey)					
100 proof	1 fl oz	0	0	0	82
	1½ fl oz	0	0	0	124
94 proof	1 fl oz	0	0	0	76
	1½ fl oz	0	0	0	116
gin, 90 proof	1½ fl oz	0	0	0	110
rum, 80 proof	1½ fl oz	0	0	0	97
vodka, 80 proof	1½ fl oz	0	0	0	97
whiskey, 86 proof	1½ fl oz	0	0	0	105
WINES					
dessert wine, sweet, 18.8% alcohol by volume	1 fl oz	0	0	0	46
table wine, 11½% alcohol by volume					
red	1 fl oz	0	0	0	21
	3½ fl oz	0	0	0	74
rosé	1 fl oz	0	0	0	21
	3½ fl oz	0	0	0	73
white	1 fl oz	0	0	0	20
	3½ fl oz	0	0	0	70

Beverages, Carbonated

Carbonated beverages contain virtually no cholesterol or fat.

Coffee & Coffee Substitutes

	Portion	Chol (mg)	Total Fat (g)	Satur'd Fat (g)	Total Calor
coffee, brewed	6 fl oz	0	0	tr	4
coffee, instant, regular or decaffeinated, powder, prepared w/water	6 fl oz water + 1 rounded t powder	0	0	tr	4
coffee substitute, cereal grain beverage, powder					
prepared w/water	6 fl oz water + 1 t powder	0	tr	tr	9
prepared w/whole milk	6 fl oz milk + 1 t powder	25	6	4	121

	Portion	Chol (mg)	Total Fat (g)	Satur'd Fat (g)	Total Calor
Flavored Milk Beverages					
carob-flavored mix					
powder	3 t	0	0	tr	45
powder, prepared w/ whole milk	1 c milk + 3 t powder	33	8	5	195
chocolate dairy drink, re- duced-calorie, aspar- tame-sweetened, powder, prepared w/ water	½ c water + 3 ice cubes + ¾ oz pkt	?	1	tr	64
chocolate-flavored mix					
powder	2–3 heap- ing t	0	1	tr	75
powder, prepared w/ whole milk	1 c milk + 2–3 heap- ing t pow- der	33	9	5	226
chocolate milk					
whole	1 c	30	8	5	208
low-fat, 2%	1 c	17	5	4	179
low-fat, 1%	1 c	7	3	2	158
chocolate syrup					
w/added nutrients	1 T	0	tr	tr	46
prepared w/whole milk	1 c milk + 1 T syrup	33	8	5	196
w/out added nutrients	1 fl oz	0	tr	tr	82
prepared w/whole milk	1 c milk + 2 T syrup	33	9	5	232
cocoa, homemade, w/	6 fl oz	24	7	4	164
whole milk	1 c	33	9	6	218
cocoa mix					
reduced-calorie, aspar- tame-sweetened, pow- der, prepared w/water	6 fl oz water + .53 oz pkt	?	tr	tr	48
w/added nutrients	6 fl oz water + 1 pkt	?	3	2	120
w/out added nutrients	6 fl oz water + 3–4 heap- ing t pow- der	?	1	1	103
eggnog, dairy	1 c	149	19	11	342
eggnog-flavored mix, pow- der, prepared w/whole milk	1 c milk + 2 heaping t powder	33	8	5	260
malt beverage	12 fl oz	0	0	0	32

	Portion	Chol (mg)	Total Fat (g)	Satur'd Fat (g)	Total Calor
malted milk–flavored mix, chocolate					
w/added nutrients					
powder	¾ oz or 4–5 heaping t	?	1	tr	75
powder, prepared w/ whole milk	1 c milk + 4–5 heaping t powder	33	9	5	225
w/out added nutrients					
powder	¾ oz or 3 heaping t	1	1	tr	79
powder, prepared w/ whole milk	1 c milk + 3 heaping t powder	34	9	6	229
malted milk–flavored mix, natural					
w/added nutrients					
powder	¾ oz or 4–5 heaping t	?	1	tr	80
powder, prepared w/ whole milk	1 c milk + 4–5 heaping t powder	33	9	5	230
w/out added nutrients					
powder	¾ oz or 3 heaping t	4	2	1	87
powder, prepared w/ whole milk	1 c milk + 3 heaping t powder	37	10	6	237
shake, thick					
chocolate	10 oz	30	8	5	335
vanilla	10 oz	33	9	5	315
strawberry-flavored mix, powder, prepared w/ whole milk	1 c milk + 2–3 heaping t powder	33	8	5	234

Fruit & Vegetable Juices

all types	1 serving	0	0 or tr	0 or tr	varies

Fruit Juice Drinks (10–50% Fruit Juice), Juice Ades, & Juice-flavored Drinks & Powders

all types	1 serving	0	0 or tr	0 or tr	varies

	Portion	Chol (mg)	Total Fat (g)	Satur'd Fat (g)	Total Calor
Tea					
brewed	6 fl oz	0	0	0	2
herb, brewed	6 fl oz	0	0	0	1
iced, canned, sweetened	12 fl oz	0	0	0	146
instant, powder					
low-cal, sodium-saccharin-sweetened, lemon-flavored	2 t	0	0	0	5
sugar-sweetened, lemon-flavored	3 rounded t	0	tr	tr	87
sweetened	3 t in 8 fl oz water	0	tr	tr	86
unsweetened	1 t	0	0	0	2
unsweetened, lemon-flavored	1 rounded t	0	0	0	4
Water					
municipal	1 c	0	0	0	0

- **BRAND NAME**

	Portion	Chol (mg)	Total Fat (g)	Satur'd Fat (g)	Total Calor
Featherweight					
hot cocoa, low-cal	6 oz	?	0	?	40
Hershey					
chocolate-flavored syrup	2 T	0	1	0	80
chocolate milk, 2% low-fat	1 c	?	5	?	190
cocoa	⅓ c	1	4	2	120
instant cocoa	3 T	0	1	0	80
International Coffees					
SUGAR-FREE					
Cafe Amaretto	6 fl oz	0	3	?	35
Cafe Français	6 fl oz	0	2	?	35
Cafe Irish Creme	6 fl oz	0	2	?	30
Cafe Vienna	6 fl oz	0	2	?	30
Irish Mocha Mint	6 fl oz	0	2	?	25
Orange Cappuccino	6 fl oz	0	2	?	30
Suisse Mocha	6 fl oz	0	2	?	30
SWEETENED W/SUGAR					
Cafe Amaretto	6 fl oz	0	2	?	50
Cafe Français	6 fl oz	0	3	?	50
Cafe Irish Creme	6 fl oz	0	3	?	60
Cafe Vienna	6 fl oz	0	2	?	60
Double Dutch Chocolate	6 fl oz	0	2	?	50
Irish Mocha Mint	6 fl oz	0	2	?	50
Orange Cappuccino	6 fl oz	0	2	?	60
Suisse Mocha	6 fl oz	0	2	?	50

	Portion	Chol (mg)	Total Fat (g)	Satur'd Fat (g)	Total Calor
Land O'Lakes					
chocolate milk					
homogenized	8 fl oz	30	8	5	210
1% low-fat	8 fl oz	5	3	2	160
skim	8 fl oz	5	<1	<1	140
eggnog	8 fl oz	123	15	10	300
Ovaltine Drink Mixes					
chocolate & malt	¾ oz dry mix	tr	tr	?	80
	¾ oz dry mix + 8 oz 2% milk	20	5	?	200
cocoa					
Hot 'n Rich	1 oz or 5 t	?	3	?	120
50-calorie	0.45 oz or about 2½ t	?	2	?	50
sugar-free	0.41 oz or about 2½ t	?	1	?	40
PDQ Drink Mixes					
chocolate	3–4 t + 8 oz whole milk	?	5	?	180
eggnog	2–3 t + 8 oz whole milk	?	5	?	230
strawberry	3–4 t + 8 oz whole milk	?	5	?	180
Perrier					
water, bottled	1 c	0	0	0	0
Poland Spring					
water, bottled	1 c	0	0	0	0
Postum					
instant hot beverage, regular or coffee-flavored	6 fl oz	0	0	0	12
Sunrise					
flavored instant coffee	0.07 oz + 6 fl oz water	?	tr	?	6

❑ **BISCUITS** *See* **BREADS, ROLLS, BISCUITS, & MUFFINS**

	Portion	Chol (mg)	Total Fat (g)	Satur'd Fat (g)	Total Calor

❑ BREADCRUMBS, CROUTONS, STUFFINGS, & SEASONED COATINGS

breadcrumbs					
enriched, dry, grated	1 c	5	5	2	390
white bread, enriched, soft	1 c	0	2	1	120
bread cubes, white, enriched	1 c	0	1	tr	80
cornflake crumbs	1 oz	0	0	0	110
croutons, herb-seasoned	0.7 oz	?	0	0	70
stuffing, from mix					
bread	½ c	?	12	?	198
corn bread	½ c	?	23	?	117
enriched bread					
dry type	1 c	0	31	6	500
moist type	1 c	67	26	5	420

▪ BRAND NAME

Kellogg's					
cornflake crumbs	1 oz	?	0	?	110
Croutettes	0.7 oz dry	?	0	?	70
Nabisco					
cracker meal	2 T	?	0	0	50
Pepperidge Farm					
croutons	½ c	?	3	?	70
stuffings	1 oz	?	1	?	110
Pillsbury Stuffing Originals					
all	½ c	?	8	?	150–170
Rice-A-Roni Stuffing Mixes					
bread/chicken flavor w/ rice, prepared	½ c	?	16	?	240
bread/herb & butter & wild rice, prepared	½ c	?	16	?	240
bread w/wild rice, prepared	½ c	?	16	?	240
corn bread w/rice, prepared	½ c	?	16	?	240
Shake 'n Bake Seasoned Coatings					
Country Milk Recipe	¼ pouch	0	4	?	80
Extra Crispy					
for chicken	¼ pouch	0	2	?	110
for pork	¼ pouch	0	3	?	120
Homestyle for chicken	¼ pouch	0	2	?	80

	Portion	Chol (mg)	Total Fat (g)	Satur'd Fat (g)	Total Calor
Stove Top					
FLEXIBLE SERVING STUFFING MIX					
chicken flavor, w/salted butter	½ c	15	9	?	170
corn bread flavor, w/salted butter	½ c	15	8	?	170
Homestyle herb, w/salted butter	½ c	15	9	?	170
STUFFING MIX					
Americana New England, w/salted butter	½ c	20	9	?	180
Americana San Francisco, w/salted butter	½ c	20	9	?	170
beef, w/salted butter	½ c	20	9	?	180
chicken flavor, w/salted butter	½ c	20	9	?	180
corn bread, w/salted butter	½ c	20	9	?	170
long grain & wild rice, w/ salted butter	½ c	20	9	?	180
savory herbs, w/salted butter	½ c	20	9	?	180
turkey, w/salted butter	½ c	20	9	?	170
wild rice, w/salted butter	½ c	20	9	?	180

❑ BREADS, ROLLS, BISCUITS, & MUFFINS

Biscuits

	Portion	Chol (mg)	Total Fat (g)	Satur'd Fat (g)	Total Calor
baking powder, prepared w/vegetable shortening					
from mix	1 (2″ diam)	tr	3	1	95
from refrigerator dough	1 (2″ diam)	1	2	1	65
homemade	1 (2″ diam)	tr	5	1	100
buttermilk, from refrigerator dough	2	?	6	?	130
flaky, from refrigerator dough	2	?	9	?	180

Bread & Bread Sticks

	Portion	Chol (mg)	Total Fat (g)	Satur'd Fat (g)	Total Calor
Boston brown bread, canned	1.6 oz slice	3	1	tr	95
bread sticks					
regular	1	?	tr	?	23
garlic	1	?	tr	?	24
sesame	1	?	4	?	56

	Portion	Chol (mg)	Total Fat (g)	Satur'd Fat (g)	Total Calor
Vienna	1	?	tr	?	18
coffee cake *See* DESSERTS: CAKES, PASTRIES, & PIES					
corn bread					
from mix	2 oz	?	4	?	160
homemade					
w/enriched cornmeal	2.9 oz	?	7	?	198
w/whole-ground corn-meal	2.7 oz	?	7	?	172
cracked-wheat bread	1 lb loaf	0	16	3	1,190
	0.9 oz slice	0	1	tr	65
danish *See* DESSERTS: CAKES, PASTRIES, & PIES					
French bread	1 lb loaf	0	18	4	1,270
	1.2 oz slice	0	1	tr	100
fruit & nut quick bread, from mix	1.4 oz slice	?	2	?	118
honey wheatberry bread	1 oz slice	?	1	?	70
Italian bread	1 lb loaf	0	4	1	1,255
	1 oz slice	0	tr	tr	85
matzo *See* CRACKERS					
mixed-grain bread	1 lb loaf	0	17	3	1,165
	0.9 oz slice	0	1	tr	65
oatmeal bread	1 lb loaf	0	20	4	1,145
	0.9 oz slice	0	1	tr	65
pita bread, white	1 piece (6½" diam)	0	1	tr	165
pumpernickel bread	1 lb loaf	0	16	3	1,160
	1.1 oz slice	0	1	tr	80
raisin bread	1 lb loaf	0	18	4	1,260
	0.9 oz slice	0	1	tr	65
roman meal bread	1 oz slice	?	1	?	68
rye bread, light	1 lb loaf	0	17	3	1,190
	0.9 oz slice	0	1	tr	65
sourdough bread	1 oz slice	?	1	?	68
Vienna bread	1 lb loaf	0	18	4	1,270
	0.9 oz slice	0	1	tr	70
wheat bread	1 lb loaf	0	19	4	1,160
	0.9 oz slice	0	1	tr	65
wheatberry bread	1 oz slice	?	1	?	70
white bread	1 lb loaf	0	18	6	1,210
	0.9 oz slice	0	1	tr	65
	0.7 oz slice	0	1	tr	55
whole-wheat bread	1 lb loaf	0	20	6	1,110
	1 oz slice	0	1	tr	70

Muffins

	Portion	Chol (mg)	Total Fat (g)	Satur'd Fat (g)	Total Calor
blueberry					
from mix	1.6 oz	45	5	1	140
homemade	1.6 oz	19	5	2	135

	Portion	Chol (mg)	Total Fat (g)	Satur'd Fat (g)	Total Calor
bran					
from mix	1.6 oz	28	4	1	140
homemade	1.6 oz	24	6	1	125
corn					
from mix	1.6 oz	42	6	2	145
homemade	1.6 oz	23	5	2	145
English					
regular	2 oz	0	1	tr	140
sourdough	2 oz	0	1	?	129

Rolls & Bagels

	Portion	Chol (mg)	Total Fat (g)	Satur'd Fat (g)	Total Calor
bagel					
plain or water, enriched	1 (3½″ diam)	0	2	tr	200
egg	1 (3½″ diam)	44	2	tr	200
brown & serve roll	1	?	2	?	92
butterflake roll, from refrigerator dough	1	?	3	?	110
buttermilk roll, from mix	1	?	5	?	113
crescent roll, from refrigerator dough	2	?	10	?	200
croissant	2 oz	13	12	4	235
dinner roll					
commercial	1 oz	tr	2	1	85
homemade	1.2 oz	12	3	1	120
frankfurter or hamburger roll	1.4 oz	tr	2	1	115
French roll, enriched	1.8 oz	?	tr	?	137
hard roll, commercial	1.2 oz	tr	2	tr	155
hoagie or submarine roll	4.8 oz	tr	8	2	400
parkerhouse roll	0.6 oz	?	2	?	59
popover					
from mix	1 oz	?	5	?	170
homemade	1.8 oz	?	5	?	112
raisin roll	2.1 oz	?	2	?	165
rye roll	0.6 oz	?	2	?	55
dark, hard	1 oz	?	1	?	80
light, hard	1 oz	?	1	?	79
sandwich roll	1.8 oz	?	3	?	162
sesame seed roll	0.6 oz	?	2	?	59
sweet roll See DESSERTS: CAKES, PASTRIES, & PIES					
wheat roll	0.6 oz	?	2	?	52
white roll					
from mix	2.2 oz	?	4	?	190
from refrigerator dough	1 oz	?	1	?	90
homemade	1.2 oz	?	3	?	119
whole-wheat roll, homemade	1.2 oz	?	1	?	90

	Portion	Chol (mg)	Total Fat (g)	Satur'd Fat (g)	Total Calor
Tortillas					
taco/tostada shell, corn	0.4 oz	?	2	?	50
tortilla, corn	1.1 oz	0	1	tr	65
canned	1.2 oz	?	1	?	75
tortilla, flour	1.1 oz	?	2	?	95

■ BRAND NAME

	Portion	Chol (mg)	Total Fat (g)	Satur'd Fat (g)	Total Calor
Lender's Bagels					
egg bagels	1	5	1	?	150
all others	1	0	0–1	?	150–160
Ortega					
taco/tostada shells	1	?	2	?	50
Pepperidge Farm					
BREADS					
cinnamon	2 slices	?	5	?	170
cracked-wheat	2 slices	?	2	?	140
Dijon rye	2 slices	?	2	?	160
Family pumpernickel	2 slices	?	2	?	160
honey bran	2 slices	?	2	?	190
honey wheatberry	2 slices	?	2	?	140
multigrain, very thin	2 slices	?	1	?	80
oatmeal	2 slices	?	3	?	140
Party Dijon Slices	4 slices	?	1	?	70
Party Pumpernickel Slices	4 slices	?	1	?	70
Party Rye Slices	4 slices	?	1	?	60
raisin w/cinnamon	2 slices	?	3	?	150
Sandwich White	2 slices	?	2	?	130
seeded Family rye	2 slices	?	1	?	80
seedless rye	2 slices	?	2	?	160
Toasting White	2 slices	?	2	?	170
wheat	2 slices	?	3	?	190
wheat germ	2 slices	?	1	?	130
white	2 slices	?	3	?	145
white, very thin	2 slices	?	1	?	80
whole-wheat	2 slices	?	2	?	130
whole-wheat, very thin	2 slices	?	2	?	80
ENGLISH MUFFINS					
plain	1	?	2	?	140
cinnamon raisin	1	?	2	?	150

	Portion	Chol (mg)	Total Fat (g)	Satur'd Fat (g)	Total Calor
OLD FASHIONED MUFFINS, FROZEN					
blueberry	1	?	6	?	170
bran w/raisins	1	?	6	?	170
carrot walnut	1	?	6	?	200
chocolate chip	1	?	8	?	210
cinnamon swirl	1	?	6	?	190
corn	1	?	7	?	180
ROLLS					
butter crescent	1	?	6	?	110
club, brown & serve	1	?	1	?	100
French style	1	?	1	?	110
golden twist	1	?	6	?	110
hamburger	1	?	2	?	130
onion sandwich buns w/ poppy seeds	1	?	3	?	150
parkerhouse	1	?	1	?	60
sourdough-style French	1	?	1	?	100
Pillsbury					
all biscuits	2	?	1–15	?	varies
bread sticks, soft	1	?	2	?	100
dinner rolls					
butterflake	1	?	4	?	110
crescent	2	?	11	?	200
sweet rolls; turnovers *See* DESSERTS: CAKES, PASTRIES, & PIES					
Sara Lee					
BAGELS					
plain	1	?	1	?	230
cinnamon & raisin	1	?	2	?	240
egg	1	?	2	?	240
onion	1	?	1	?	220
poppy seed	1	?	1	?	230
HEARTY FRUIT MUFFINS					
apple cinnamon spice	1	?	8	?	220
banana nut bran	1	?	9	?	230
blueberry	1	?	8	?	200
oatmeal & fruit	1	?	9	?	230
L'ORIGINAL CROISSANTS					
all butter	1	?	9	?	170
petite size	1	?	6	?	120
presliced	1	?	9	?	170
cheese	1	?	9	?	170
wheat & honey	1	?	9	?	170

	Portion	Chol (mg)	Total Fat (g)	Satur'd Fat (g)	Total Calor

LE PASTRIE CROISSANTS See DESSERTS: CAKES, PASTRIES, & PIES

LE SANDWICH CROISSANTS See ENTREES & MAIN COURSES, FROZEN

❑ BREAKFAST CEREALS, COLD & HOT

Cold Cereal

	Portion	Chol (mg)	Total Fat (g)	Satur'd Fat (g)	Total Calor
cornflakes, low-sodium	1 oz or about 1 c	?	tr	?	113
crisp rice, low-sodium	1 oz or about 1 c	?	tr	?	114
granola, homemade	1 oz or about ¼ c	?	8	1	138
	1 c	?	33	6	595
oat flakes, fortified	1 oz or about ⅔ c	?	tr	?	105
	1 c	?	1	?	177
rice, puffed	½ oz or about 1 c	?	tr	?	57
wheat, puffed, plain	½ oz or about 1 c (heaping)	?	tr	?	52
wheat, shredded large biscuit	1 rectangular	?	tr	?	83
	2 round	?	1	?	133
small biscuit	1 oz or about ⅔ c	?	1	?	102
	⅞ oz box	?	1	?	89
wheat germ, toasted plain	1 oz or about ¼ c	?	3	1	108
	1 c	?	12	2	431
w/brown sugar & honey	1 oz or about ¼ c	?	2	tr	107
	1 c	?	9	2	426

Hot Cereal

	Portion	Chol (mg)	Total Fat (g)	Satur'd Fat (g)	Total Calor
corn grits regular & quick dry	1 c	?	2	?	579
	1 T	?	tr	?	36
cooked	1 c	?	1	?	146
	¾ c	?	tr	?	110

	Portion	Chol (mg)	Total Fat (g)	Satur'd Fat (g)	Total Calor
corn grits *(cont.)*					
instant, prepared					
plain	1 pkt	?	tr	?	82
w/artificial cheese flavor	1 pkt	?	1	?	107
w/imitation bacon bits	1 pkt	?	1	?	104
w/imitation ham bits	1 pkt	?	tr	?	103
farina					
dry	1 c	?	1	?	649
	1 T	?	tr	?	40
cooked	1 c	?	tr	?	116
	¾ c	?	tr	?	87
grits; hominy grits *See* corn grits, *above*					
oats, regular, quick, & instant, nonfortified					
dry	⅓ c	?	2	tr	104
cooked	1 c	?	2	tr	145
	¾ c	?	2	tr	108

▪ BRAND NAME

Arrowhead Mills
COLD CEREAL

	Portion	Chol (mg)	Total Fat (g)	Satur'd Fat (g)	Total Calor
Agrain & Agrain	2 oz	0	2	?	220
Arrowhead Crunch	1 oz	0	3	?	120
bran flakes	1 oz	0	1	?	100
corn, puffed	½ oz	0	0	?	50
cornflakes	1 oz	0	1	?	110
granola					
apple amaranth	2 oz	0	6	?	225
maple nut	2 oz	0	11	?	260
millet, puffed	½ oz	0	0	?	50
Nature O's	1 oz	0	1	?	110
rice, puffed	½ oz	0	0	?	50
wheat, puffed	½ oz	0	0	?	50
wheat bran	2 oz	0	2	?	200
wheat germ, raw	2 oz	0	6	?	210

HOT CEREAL

	Portion	Chol (mg)	Total Fat (g)	Satur'd Fat (g)	Total Calor
Bear Mush	1 oz	0	0	?	100
corn grits, white or yellow	2 oz	0	1	?	200
4 Grain & Flax	2 oz	0	1	?	94
oat bran	1 oz	0	2	?	110
oatmeal, instant	1 oz	0	2	?	100
oats, steel cut	2 oz	0	4	?	220
Rice & Shine	¼ c	0	1	?	160
Seven Grain	1 oz	0	1	?	100
wheat, cracked	2 oz	0	1	?	180

	Portion	Chol (mg)	Total Fat (g)	Satur'd Fat (g)	Total Calor
Erewhon					
COLD CEREAL					
Crispy Brown Rice, regular or low-sodium	1 oz or about 1 c	0	1	?	110
Fruit 'n Wheat	1 oz or about ½ c	0	1	?	100
granola					
date nut	1 oz or about ¼ c	0	6	?	130
honey almond	1 oz or about ¼ c	0	6	?	130
maple	1 oz or about ¼ c	0	5	?	130
#9, w/bran, no salt added	1 oz or about ¼ c	0	6	?	130
spiced apple	1 oz or about ¼ c	0	6	?	130
Sunflower Crunch	1 oz or about ¼ c	0	4	?	130
raisin bran	1 oz or about ½ c	0	0	?	100
wheat flakes	1 oz or about ½ c	0	0	?	110
HOT CEREAL					
Barley Plus	1 oz or about ⅓ c dry	0	1	?	110
brown rice cream	1 oz or about ⅓ c dry	0	1	?	110
oat bran w/toasted wheat germ	1 oz or about ⅓ c dry	0	2	?	115
Featherweight Cold Cereal					
cornflakes	1¼ c	?	0	?	110
General Mills Cold Cereal					
Cheerios					
regular	1 oz or about 1¼ c	?	2	tr	111
	¾ oz box	?	1	tr	83
Honey Nut	1 oz or about ¾ c	?	1	tr	107
	1 c	?	1	tr	125
Crispy Wheats 'n Raisins	1 oz or about ¾ c	?	1	?	99
	1 c	?	1	?	150

	Portion	Chol (mg)	Total Fat (g)	Satur'd Fat (g)	Total Calor
Golden Grahams	1 oz or about ¾ c	?	1	1	109
	1 c	?	2	1	150
Kix	1 oz or about 1½ c	?	1	tr	110
	¾ oz box	?	1	tr	83
Lucky Charms	1 oz or about 1 c	?	1	tr	110
Total	1 oz or about 1 c	?	1	tr	100
Trix	1 oz or about 1 c	?	tr	?	109
Wheaties	1 oz or about 1 c	?	1	tr	99

Health Valley
COLD CEREAL

	Portion	Chol (mg)	Total Fat (g)	Satur'd Fat (g)	Total Calor
Amaranth Crunch w/raisins	1 oz or about ¼ c	0	3	?	110
amaranth flakes	1 oz or about ½ c	0	1	?	110
amaranth w/banana	1 oz or about ¼ c	0	2	?	100
bran, w/apples & cinnamon or w/raisins	1 oz or about ¼ c	0	1	?	100
Fiber 7 Flakes	1 oz or about ½ c	0	1	?	100
Fruit Lites					
corn	½ oz or about ½ c	0	0	?	43
rice	½ oz or about ½ c	0	0	?	45
wheat	½ oz or about ½ c	0	0	?	43
granola See Real Granola, below					
Healthy Crunch, w/almonds & dates or w/ apples & cinnamon	1 oz or about ¼ c	0	3	?	120
Lites, corn, rice, or wheat, puffed	½ oz or about ½ c	0	0	?	50
oat bran flakes					
plain or w/almonds & dates	1 oz or about ½ c	0	2	?	110
w/raisins	1 oz or about ½ c	0	1	?	107
Orangeola, w/almonds & dates or w/banana & Hawaiian fruit	1 oz or about ¼ c	0	4	?	120
raisin bran flakes	1 oz or about ½ c	0	0	?	110

	Portion	Chol (mg)	Total Fat (g)	Satur'd Fat (g)	Total Calor
Real Granola, w/almond crunch, w/Hawaiian fruit, or w/raisins & nuts	1 oz or about ¼ c	0	3	?	120
Sprouts 7, w/bananas & Hawaiian fruit or w/raisins	1 oz or about ¼ c	0	1	?	100
stoned-wheat flakes	1 oz or about ⅔ c	0	0	?	110
Swiss Breakfast, raisin nut or tropical fruit	1 oz or about ¼ c	0	2	?	100
wheat bran/Millers Flakes	2 oz	0	3	?	121
wheat germ w/fiber, almonds & dates or bananas & tropical fruit	1 oz or about ¼ c	0	1	?	100

HOT CEREAL

hot oat bran w/apples	1 oz or ¼ c	0	1	?	110

Heartland Cold Cereal
Natural Cereal

plain	1 oz or about ¼ c	?	4	?	123
	1 c	?	18	?	499
w/coconut	1 oz or about ¼ c	?	5	?	125
	1 c	?	17	?	463
w/raisins	1 oz or about ¼ c	?	4	?	120
	1 c	?	16	?	467

Kellogg's Cold Cereal

All-Bran	1 oz or about ⅓ c	0	1	?	70
w/extra fiber	1 oz or about ½ c	0	1	?	60
w/fruit & almonds	1.3 oz or about ⅔ c	0	2	?	100
Apple Jacks	1 oz or about 1 c	0	0	?	110
Bran Buds	1 oz or about ⅓ c	0	1	?	70
bran flakes	1 oz or about ⅔ c	0	0	?	90
Cocoa Krispies	1 oz or about ¾ c	0	0	?	110
Corn Flakes regular	1 oz or about 1 c	0	0	?	110
honey & nut	1 oz or about ⅔ c	0	1	?	110

	Portion	Chol (mg)	Total Fat (g)	Satur'd Fat (g)	Total Calor
Corn Pops	1 oz or about 1 c	0	0	?	110
Cracklin' Oat Bran	1 oz or about ½ c	0	4	?	110
Crispix	1 oz or about 1 c	0	0	?	110
Froot Loops	1 oz or about 1 c	0	1	?	110
Frosted Flakes	1 oz or about ¾ c	0	0	?	110
Frosted Krispies	1 oz or about ¾ c	0	0	?	110
Frosted Mini-Wheats	1 oz = about 4 biscuits	0	0	?	100
Fruitful Bran	1.3 oz or about ⅔ c	0	0	?	120
Honey Smacks	1 oz or about ¾ c	0	0	?	110
Just Right					
all-grain	1 oz or about ⅔ c	0	0	?	100
w/fruit	1.3 oz or about ¾ c	0	1	?	140
Nutri-Grain					
almond raisin	1.4 oz or about ⅔ c	0	2	?	150
corn	1 oz or about ½ c	0	1	?	100
wheat	1 oz or about ⅔ c	0	0	?	100
wheat & raisins	1.4 oz or about ⅔ c	0	0	?	130
Product 19	1 oz or about 1 c	0	0	?	110
raisin bran	1.4 oz or about ¾ c	0	1	?	120
Rice Krispies	1 oz or about 1 c	0	0	?	110
Special K	1 oz or about 1 c	0	0	?	110
Maltex Hot Cereal					
Maltex					
dry	¼ c	?	1	?	134
cooked	1 c	?	1	?	180
	¾ c	?	1	?	135
Old Fashioned Maltex	½ c cooked	0	tr	?	77

	Portion	Chol (mg)	Total Fat (g)	Satur'd Fat (g)	Total Calor
Malt-O-Meal Hot Cereal					
Malt-O-Meal, plain or chocolate					
dry	1 T	?	tr	?	38
cooked	1 c	?	tr	?	122
	¾ c	?	tr	?	92
Maypo					
Maypo					
dry	½ c	?	3	?	181
cooked	1 c	?	2	?	170
	¾ c	?	2	?	128
30-Second Oatmeal					
regular	½ c cooked	0	1	?	89
maple flavor	1 oz dry	0	1	?	101
Vermont-Style Hot Oat Cereal	½ c cooked	0	1	?	77
Nabisco					
COLD CEREAL					
Fruit Wheats, apple, raisin, or strawberry	1 oz	?	0	?	100
100% Bran	1 oz or about ½ c	?	1	tr	76
	1 c	?	3	1	178
Shredded Wheat 'n Bran	1 oz	?	1	?	110
Team	1 oz or about 1 c	?	1	?	111
Toasted Wheat & Raisins	1 oz	?	1	?	100
HOT CEREAL					
Cream of Rice	1 oz dry	?	0	?	100
Cream of Wheat					
regular or instant	1 oz dry	?	0	?	100
Mix 'n Eat					
Original	1 oz dry	?	0	?	100
w/apple & cinnamon, w/ brown sugar cinnamon, or w/maple brown sugar	1¼ oz dry	?	0	?	130
w/peach or w/strawberry	1¼ oz dry	?	2	?	140
quick					
regular	1 oz dry	?	0	?	100
w/apples, raisins, & spice or w/maple brown sugar, artificially flavored	1 oz dry	?	1	?	110
Nature Valley Cold Cereal					
granola, toasted oat mixture	1 oz or about ⅓ c	?	5	3	126
	1 c	?	20	13	503

	Portion	Chol (mg)	Total Fat (g)	Satur'd Fat (g)	Total Calor
Post Cold Cereal					
Alpha-Bits	1 oz	0	1	?	110
Cocoa Pebbles	1 oz	0	1	?	110
C.W. Post Hearty Granola					
plain	1 oz	0	4	?	130
w/raisins	1 oz	0	4	?	120
Frosted Rice Krinkles	1 oz or about ⅞ c	?	tr	?	109
Fruit & Fibre: dates, raisins, walnuts; Harvest Medley; Mountain Trail; or tropical fruit	1 oz	0	1	?	90
Fruity Pebbles	1 oz	0	1	?	110
granola *See* C.W. Post Hearty Granola, *above*					
Grape-Nuts					
regular	1 oz	0	0	0	110
raisin	1 oz	0	0	0	100
Grape-Nuts Flakes	1 oz	0	1	?	100
Honeycomb	1 oz	0	0	0	110
Natural Bran Flakes	1 oz	0	0	0	90
Natural Raisin Bran	1 oz	0	0	0	80
oat flakes, fortified	1 oz	0	1	?	110
Post Toasties	1 oz	0	0	0	110
Super Golden Crisp	1 oz or about ⅞ c	?	0	?	110
Quaker Oats					
COLD CEREAL					
bran, unprocessed	2 T	?	tr	?	21
Cap'n Crunch					
regular	1 oz or about ¾ c	?	3	2	119
	1 c	?	3	2	156
w/Crunchberries	1 oz or about ¾ c	?	2	2	118
	1 c	?	3	2	146
peanut butter	1 oz or about ¾ c	?	4	2	124
	1 c	?	5	2	154
corn bran	1 oz or about ⅔ c	?	1	?	98
	1 c	?	1	?	124
King Vitaman	1 oz or about 1¼ c	?	2	1	115
	1 c	?	1	1	85
100% Natural Cereal					
plain	1 oz or about ¼ c	?	6	4	133
	1 c	?	22	15	489

	Portion	Chol (mg)	Total Fat (g)	Satur'd Fat (g)	Total Calor
w/apples & cinnamon	1 oz or about ¼ c	?	5	4	130
	1 c	?	20	15	478
w/raisins & dates	1 oz or about ¼ c	?	5	4	128
	1 c	?	20	14	496
Life, plain or cinnamon	1 oz or about ⅔ c	?	1	?	104
	1 c	?	1	?	162
Mr. T	1 c	?	3	?	121
Quisp	1 oz or about 1 c	?	2	1	117

HOT CEREAL

	Portion	Chol (mg)	Total Fat (g)	Satur'd Fat (g)	Total Calor
farina, quick creamy wheat	2½ T uncooked	?	0	?	101
oat bran	⅓ c uncooked	?	3	?	110
oatmeal, instant, prepared					
regular	1 pkt	?	2	?	105
w/apples & cinnamon	1 pkt	?	2	?	134
w/artificial maple & brown sugar	1 pkt	?	2	?	163
w/bran & raisins	1 pkt	?	2	?	153
w/cinnamon & spice	1 pkt	?	2	?	176
w/peaches & cream or w/ strawberries & cream, both artificially flavored	1 pkt	?	2	?	136
w/raisins & spice	1 pkt	?	2	?	159
w/raisins, dates, & walnuts	1 pkt	?	4	?	150
w/real honey & graham	1 pkt	?	2	?	136
Quaker Oats, Quick & Old Fashioned	⅓ c dry or ⅔ c cooked	?	2	?	109
Whole Wheat Hot Natural	⅓ c dry or ⅔ c cooked	?	1	?	106

Ralston Purina
COLD CEREAL

	Portion	Chol (mg)	Total Fat (g)	Satur'd Fat (g)	Total Calor
Bran Chex	1 oz or about ⅔ c	?	1	?	91
	1 c	?	1	?	156
Cookie-Crisp	1 oz or about 1 c	?	1	?	114
Corn Chex	1 oz or about 1 c	?	tr	?	111
	¾ oz box	?	tr	?	84
cornflakes	1 oz or about 1 c	?	tr	?	111

	Portion	Chol (mg)	Total Fat (g)	Satur'd Fat (g)	Total Calor
40% bran flakes	1 oz or about ¾ c	?	tr	?	92
	1 c	?	1	?	159
raisin bran	1⅓ oz or about ¾ c	?	tr	?	120
	1 c	?	tr	?	178
Rice Chex	1 oz or about 1⅛ c	?	tr	?	112
	⅞ oz box	?	tr	?	98
sugar frosted flakes	1 oz or about ¾ c	?	tr	?	111
	1 c	?	1	?	149
Tasteeos	1 oz or about 1¼ c	?	1	?	111
	1 c	?	1	?	94
Waffelos	1 oz or about 1 c	?	1	?	115
Wheat Chex	1 oz or about ⅔ c	?	1	?	104
	1 c	?	1	?	169
Wheat 'n Raisin Chex	1⅓ oz or about ¾ c	?	tr	?	130
	1 c	?	tr	?	185

HOT CEREAL

	Portion	Chol (mg)	Total Fat (g)	Satur'd Fat (g)	Total Calor
Ralston					
dry	¼ c	?	1	?	102
cooked	1 c	?	1	?	134
	¾ c	?	1	?	100

Roman Meal Hot Cereal

	Portion	Chol (mg)	Total Fat (g)	Satur'd Fat (g)	Total Calor
Roman Meal					
plain					
dry	⅓ c	?	1	?	100
cooked	1 c	?	1	?	147
	¾ c	?	1	?	111
w/oats					
dry	¼ c	?	1	?	85
cooked	1 c	?	2	?	169
	¾ c	?	2	?	127

Sun Country Granola

	Portion	Chol (mg)	Total Fat (g)	Satur'd Fat (g)	Total Calor
w/almonds	1 oz	0	5	?	130
w/raisins	1 oz	0	5	?	130
w/raisins & dates	1 oz	0	4	?	130

Sunshine

	Portion	Chol (mg)	Total Fat (g)	Satur'd Fat (g)	Total Calor
shredded wheat					
regular	1 biscuit	0	1	?	90
bite size	⅔ c	0	1	?	110

	Portion	Chol (mg)	Total Fat (g)	Satur'd Fat (g)	Total Calor
U.S. Mills See also Erewhon, *above*					
Skinner's raisin bran	1 oz or about ½ c	0	1	?	100
Uncle Sam, laxative	1 oz or about ½ c	0	2	?	110
Wheatena Hot Cereal					
Wheatena					
dry	¼ c	?	1	?	125
cooked	1 c	?	1	?	135
	¾ c	?	1	?	101

❑ BREAKFAST FOODS, PREPARED

See also EGGS & EGG SUBSTITUTES; FAST FOODS

	Portion	Chol (mg)	Total Fat (g)	Satur'd Fat (g)	Total Calor
French toast, homemade	1 slice	112	7	2	155
pancakes					
from mix					
plain	1 (4″ diam)	16	2	1	60
buckwheat	1 (4″ diam)	20	2	1	55
extra light	3 (4″ diam)	?	7	?	200
homemade					
plain	1 (4″ diam)	16	2	1	60
cornmeal	1 (4″ diam)	?	1	?	68
soy	1 (4″ diam)	?	2	?	68
waffles					
from mix	1 (7″ diam)	59	8	3	205
frozen	1	?	3	?	95
homemade	1 (7″ diam)	102	13	4	245

▪ BRAND NAME

	Portion	Chol (mg)	Total Fat (g)	Satur'd Fat (g)	Total Calor
Arrowhead Mills Pancake Mixes					
Blue Heaven	½ c	tr	2	?	200
buckwheat	½ c	tr	2	?	270
Griddle Lite	½ c	tr	3	?	260
multigrain	½ c	tr	2	?	350
triticale	½ c	tr	2	?	270
Aunt Jemima					
FRENCH TOAST, FROZEN					
plain	2 slices	?	4	?	168
cinnamon swirl	2 slices	?	6	?	190
raisin	2 slices	?	4	?	185
PANCAKE & WAFFLE MIXES					
original flavor	¼ c	?	1	?	108
buckwheat	¼ c	?	1	?	107

	Portion	Chol (mg)	Total Fat (g)	Satur'd Fat (g)	Total Color
buttermilk	⅓ c	?	1	?	175
whole-wheat	⅓ c	?	1	?	142
PANCAKE BATTER, FROZEN					
original flavor	3 (4″ diam)	?	2	?	210
blueberry	3 (4″ diam)	?	2	?	205
buttermilk	3 (4″ diam)	?	2	?	212
PANCAKES, FROZEN					
original flavor	3 (4″ diam)	?	4	?	246
blueberry	3 (4″ diam)	?	4	?	249
buttermilk	3 (4″ diam)	?	4	?	240
WAFFLES, FROZEN					
original flavor	2	?	4	?	173
apple & cinnamon	2	?	4	?	173
blueberry	2	?	4	?	173
buttermilk	2	?	4	?	175
Fearn Pancake Mixes					
buckwheat	½ c dry	0	3	tr	235
Rich Earth	½ c dry	0	2	tr	190
7-grain buttermilk	½ c dry	1	2	1	200
stone-ground whole-wheat	½ c dry	0	2	tr	220
unbleached wheat & soya	½ c dry	0	2	tr	235
Featherweight					
pancake mix	3 (4″ diam)	?	1	?	130
Health Valley					
7 Sprouted Grains buttermilk pancake & biscuit mix	1 oz	0	1	?	100
Kellogg's					
EGGO FROZEN WAFFLES					
apple cinnamon	1	?	5	?	130
buttermilk	1	?	5	?	120
Homestyle	1	?	5	?	120
POP-TARTS See DESSERTS: CAKES, PASTRIES, & PIES					
Nabisco Toastettes *See* DESSERTS: CAKES, PASTRIES, & PIES					
Swanson					
GREAT STARTS BREAKFASTS					
French toast (cinnamon swirl)	6½ oz	?	28	?	480
French toast w/sausages	6½ oz	?	27	?	460
omelets w/cheese sauce & ham	7 oz	?	31	?	400
pancakes & blueberry sauce	7 oz	?	10	?	410
pancakes & sausages	6 oz	?	22	?	470

	Portion	Chol (mg)	Total Fat (g)	Satur'd Fat (g)	Total Calor
scrambled eggs & sausage w/hashed brown pota toes	6¼ oz	?	34	?	430
Spanish-style omelet	7¾ oz	?	17	?	250
GREAT STARTS BREAKFAST SANDWICHES					
biscuit & sausage	4¾ oz	?	23	?	410
egg, Canadian bacon, & cheese/muffin	4½ oz	?	16	?	310
sausage, egg, & cheese/ biscuit	6¼ oz	?	32	?	520
steak, egg, & cheese/ muffin	5¼ oz	?	23	?	390

❏ BROWNIES *See* COOKIES, BARS, & BROWNIES

❏ BUTTER & MARGARINE SPREADS

Butter
See also NUTS & NUT-BASED BUTTERS, FLOURS, MEALS, MILKS, PASTES, & POWDERS; SEEDS & SEED-BASED BUTTERS, FLOURS, & MEALS

	Portion	Chol (mg)	Total Fat (g)	Satur'd Fat (g)	Total Calor
salted or unsalted	1 t	11	4	2½	36
	1 stick = 4 oz or about ½ c	247	92	57	813
whipped, salted	1 t	8	3	2	27
	1 stick = 4 oz or about ½ c	165	61	38	542

Margarine

REGULAR

Hard, Stick or Brick

	Portion	Chol (mg)	Total Fat (g)	Satur'd Fat (g)	Total Calor
coconut, safflower, coco nut (hydrogenated), & palm (hydrogenated)	1 stick	0	91	65	815
	1 t	0	4	3	34
corn (hydrogenated)	1 stick	0	91	15	815
	1 t	0	4	1	34
corn & corn (hydrogen- ated)	1 stick	0	91	16	815
	1 t	0	4	1	34

	Portion	Chol (mg)	Total Fat (g)	Satur'd Fat (g)	Total Calor
corn, soybean (hydrogenated), & cottonseed (hydrogenated)					
salted	1 stick	0	91	17	815
	1 t	0	4	1	34
unsalted	1 stick	0	91	17	810
	1 t	0	4	1	34
lard (hydrogenated)	1 stick	57	91	36	831
	1 t	2	4	2	35
safflower & soybean (hydrogenated)	1 stick	0	91	16	815
	1 t	0	4	1	34
safflower, soybean (hydrogenated), & cottonseed (hydrogenated)	1 stick	0	91	15	815
	1 t	0	4	1	34
safflower, soybean, soybean (hydrogenated), & cottonseed (hydrogenated)	1 stick	0	91	16	815
	1 t	0	4	1	34
soybean (hydrogenated)	1 stick	0	91	19	815
	1 t	0	4	1	34
soybean & soybean (hydrogenated)	1 stick	0	91	15	815
	1 t	0	4	1	34
soybean (hydrogenated) & cottonseed	1 stick	0	91	19	815
	1 t	0	4	1	34
soybean (hydrogenated) & cottonseed (hydrogenated)	1 stick	0	91	17	815
	1 t	0	4	1	34
soybean (hydrogenated) & palm (hydrogenated)	1 stick	0	91	17	815
	1 t	0	4	1	34
soybean (hydrogenated), corn, & cottonseed (hydrogenated)	1 stick	0	91	23	815
	1 t	0	4	1	34
soybean (hydrogenated), cottonseed (hydrogenated), & soybean	1 stick	0	91	18	815
	1 t	0	4	1	34
soybean (hydrogenated), palm (hydrogenated), & palm	1 stick	0	91	20	815
	1 t	0	4	1	34
sunflower, soybean (hydrogenated), & cottonseed (hydrogenated)	1 stick	0	91	14	815
	1 t	0	4	1	34
Liquid, Bottle					
soybean (hydrogenated), soybean, & cottonseed	1 c	0	183	30	1,637
	1 t	0	4	1	34
Soft, Tub					
corn & corn (hydrogenated)	1 c	0	183	32	1,626
	1 t	0	4	1	34

	Portion	Chol (mg)	Total Fat (g)	Satur'd Fat (g)	Total Calor
safflower, cottonseed (hydrogenated), & peanut (hydrogenated)	1 c	0	183	30	1,626
	1 t	0	4	1	34
safflower & safflower (hydrogenated)	1 c	0	183	21	1,626
	1 t	0	4	tr	34
soybean (hydrogenated)					
salted	1 c	0	183	31	1,626
	1 t	0	4	1	34
unsalted	1 c	0	182	31	1,626
	1 t	0	4	1	34
soybean (hydrogenated) & cottonseed	1 c	0	183	37	1,626
	1 t	0	4	1	34
soybean (hydrogenated) & cottonseed (hydrogenated)					
salted	1 c	0	183	32	1,626
	1 t	0	4	1	34
unsalted	1 c	0	182	32	1,626
	1 t	0	4	1	34
soybean (hydrogenated) & safflower	1 c	0	183	24	1,626
	1 t	0	4	1	34
soybean (hydrogenated), cottonseed (hydrogenated), & soybean	1 c	0	183	35	1,626
	1 t	0	4	1	34
soybean (hydrogenated), palm (hydrogenated), & palm	1 c	0	183	39	1,626
	1 t	0	4	1	34
soybean, soybean (hydrogenated), & cottonseed (hydrogenated)	1 c	0	183	37	1,626
	1 t	0	4	1	34
sunflower, cottonseed (hydrogenated), & peanut (hydrogenated)	1 c	0	183	29	1,626
	1 t	0	4	1	34

IMITATION (ABOUT 40% FAT)

	Portion	Chol (mg)	Total Fat (g)	Satur'd Fat (g)	Total Calor
corn & corn (hydrogenated)	1 c	0	90	15	801
	1 t	0	2	tr	17
soybean (hydrogenated)	1 c	0	90	15	801
	1 t	0	2	tr	17
soybean (hydrogenated) & cottonseed	1 c	0	90	19	801
	1 t	0	2	tr	17
soybean (hydrogenated) & cottonseed (hydrogenated)	1 c	0	90	17	801
	1 t	0	2	tr	17
soybean (hydrogenated), palm (hydrogenated), & palm	1 c	0	90	24	801
	1 t	0	2	1	17
unspecified ingredient oils	1 c	0	90	18	801
	1 t	0	2	tr	17

	Portion	Chol (mg)	Total Fat (g)	Satur'd Fat (g)	Total Calor
SPREAD, MARGARINELIKE (ABOUT 60% FAT)					
Stick					
soybean (hydrogenated) &	1 c	0	139	32	1,236
palm (hydrogenated)	1 t	0	3	1	26
Tub					
soybean (hydrogenated) &	1 c	0	139	28	1,236
cottonseed (hydrogenated)	1 t	0	3	1	26
soybean (hydrogenated),	1 c	0	139	31	1,236
palm (hydrogenated), & palm	1 t	0	3	1	26
unspecified ingredient oils	1 c	0	139	29	1,236
	1 t	0	3	1	26

▪ BRAND NAME

Blue Bonnet Margarine					
Butter Blend, soft or stick, salted or unsalted	1 T	5	11	2	90
margarine					
regular, soft or stick	1 T	0	11	2	100
diet	1 T	0	6	1	50
whipped, soft or stick	1 T	0	7	2	70
spread					
Light Tasty, 52% vegetable oil	1 T	0	7	1	60
52% fat	1 T	0	8	2	80
stick, 70% fat	1 T	0	10	2	90
stick, 75% fat	1 T	0	11	2	90
whipped, 60% fat	1 T	0	6	1	50
Fleischmann's					
margarine					
regular: stick, soft, or squeeze; salted or unsalted	1 T	0	11	2	100
diet or diet w/lite salt	1 T	0	6	1	50
whipped, salted or unsalted	1 T	0	7	2	70
spread, light corn oil, soft or stick	1 T	0	8	2	80
Land O'Lakes					
butter					
regular, salted or unsalted	1 T	30	11	7	100
whipped, salted or unsalted	1 T	20	7	4	60

	Portion	Chol (mg)	Total Fat (g)	Satur'd Fat (g)	Total Calor
Country Morning Blend margarine					
stick, salted or unsalted	1 T	10	11	3	100
soft, tub, salted or unsalted	1 T	10	10	3	90
margarine, stick or soft tub, regular (soy oil) or premium (corn oil)	1 T	0	11	2	100
Mazola margarine					
regular, salted or unsalted	1 T	0	11	2	100
diet	1 T	0	6	1	50
Nucoa					
soft margarine	1 T	0	10	2	90

❑ CAKES *See* DESSERTS: CAKES, PASTRIES, & PIES

❑ CANDIED FRUIT *See* BAKING INGREDIENTS

❑ CANDY

	Portion	Chol (mg)	Total Fat (g)	Satur'd Fat (g)	Total Calor
butterscotch	6 pieces	?	3	?	116
butterscotch chips	1 oz	tr	7	?	150
caramels					
plain or chocolate	3	?	3	?	112
plain or chocolate w/nuts	2	?	5	?	120
chocolate					
chocolate fudge center	1	?	5	?	129
chocolate fudge w/nuts center	1	?	6	?	127
coconut center	1	?	5	?	123
cream center	1	?	4	?	102
fondant center	1	?	3	?	115
vanilla cream center	1	?	4	?	114
chocolate chips					
chocolate-flavored	¼ c	tr	8	2	195
dark	1 oz	?	8	?	148
milk chocolate	¼ c	7	11	?	218
semisweet	1 c or 6 oz (60 chips/ oz)	0	61	36	860

	Portion	Chol (mg)	Total Fat (g)	Satur'd Fat (g)	Total Calor
chocolate-covered almonds	1 oz	?	12	?	159
chocolate-covered Brazil nuts	1 oz	?	14	?	162
chocolate-covered peanuts	1 oz	?	9	?	153
chocolate-covered raisins	1 oz	?	4	?	115
chocolate kisses	6	?	9	?	154
chocolate stars	7	?	8	?	145
English toffee	1 oz	?	17	?	193
fondant, uncoated (mints, candy corn, other)	1 oz	0	0	0	105
fudge					
chocolate, plain	1 oz	1	3	2	115
chocolate w/nuts	1 oz	?	5	?	119
vanilla	1 oz	?	3	?	111
vanilla w/nuts	1 oz	?	5	?	119
granola bars See COOKIES, BARS, & BROWNIES					
gum drops	1 oz	0	tr	tr	100
hard candy	1 oz	0	0	0	110
	6 pieces	0	tr	0	108
jelly beans	1 oz	0	tr	tr	105
	10	0	0	0	66
lollipop	1 medium	0	0	0	108
malted milk balls	14	?	7	?	135
marshmallows	1 oz	0	0	0	90
	1 large	0	0	0	25
mints	14	?	1	?	104
peanut brittle	1 oz	?	4	?	123
sugar-coated almonds	7	?	5	?	128

▪ BRAND NAME

NOTE: Candies may be listed under product name (e.g., Milky Way) or company name (e.g., Cadbury or Hershey).

	Portion	Chol (mg)	Total Fat (g)	Satur'd Fat (g)	Total Calor
Almond Joy	1 oz	?	8	?	151
Baby Ruth	½ bar	?	6	?	130
Baker's chocolate See BAKING INGREDIENTS					
Beechies candy-coated gum, all flavors	1 piece	?	0	?	6
Beech-Nut					
cough drops, all flavors	1	?	0	?	10
gum, all flavors	1 piece	?	0	?	10
Bit-O-Honey	1 oz	?	4	?	121
	1.8 oz	?	7	?	220
Bonkers!, all flavors	1 piece	?	0	?	20
Breath Savers Mints, sugar-free, all flavors	1	?	0	?	8
Bubble Yum bubble gum, all flavors					
regular	1 piece	?	0	?	25

	Portion	Chol (mg)	Total Fat (g)	Satur'd Fat (g)	Total Calor
sugarless	1 piece	?	0	?	20
Butterfinger	½ bar	?	6	?	130
Butter Nut	1.8 oz	?	12	?	250
Cadbury					
chocolate almond	1 oz	?	9	?	155
chocolate Brazil nut	1 oz	?	9	?	156
chocolate hazelnut	1 oz	?	9	?	155
chocolate Krisp	1 oz	?	7	?	146
creme eggs	1 oz	?	6	?	136
fruit & nut	1 oz	?	9	?	152
milk chocolate	1 oz	?	8	?	151
Caramello	1 oz	?	8	?	144
Caravelle	1 oz	?	5	?	137
Care-Free					
sugarless bubble gum, all flavors	1 piece	?	0	?	10
sugarless gum, all flavors	1 piece	?	0	?	8
Charleston Chew!	½ piece	?	3	?	120
Chunky					
Original	1 oz	?	7	?	143
milk chocolate	1 oz	?	4	?	120
peanut	1 oz	?	9	?	151
pecan	1 oz	?	8	?	148
Fruit Stripe					
bubble gum, all flavors	1 piece	?	0	?	10
gum, all flavors	1 piece	?	0	?	10
Good 'n Fruity	1½ oz	?	tr	?	160
Good & Plenty	1½ oz	?	tr	?	151
Hershey					
chocolate chips & unsweetened chocolate *See* BAKING INGREDIENTS					
chocolate Kisses	9 or 1.46 oz	7	13	8	220
Krackel	1.6 oz	9	14	8	250
milk chocolate	1.65 oz	12	14	9	250
milk chocolate w/almonds	1.55 oz	12	15	7	250
Special Dark sweet chocolate	1.45 oz	3	12	7	220
Junior Mints	12	?	3	?	120
Kit Kat	1.6 oz	12	13	8	250
Life Savers					
lollipops, all flavors	1	?	0	?	45
milk chocolate stars	13	?	8	?	160
roll candy, all flavors, regular or sugar-free	1 piece	?	0	?	8
M&M's					
regular	1.59 oz	?	10	?	220
peanut	1.67 oz	?	12	?	240
Marathon	1.38 oz	?	7	?	179
Mars	1.7 oz	?	10	?	230
Milk Mounds	1 oz	?	8	?	138

	Portion	Chol (mg)	Total Fat (g)	Satur'd Fat (g)	Total Calor
Milk Shake	2 oz	?	8	?	250
Milky Way	2.1 oz	?	9	?	260
Mounds	1 oz	?	7	?	147
Mr. Goodbar	1.85 oz	12	20	8	300
Nestlé					
Crunch	1.06 oz	5	8	?	160
milk chocolate	1.07 oz	?	9	?	160
milk chocolate w/ almonds	1 oz	5	9	?	150
Oh Henry!	1 oz	?	7	?	139
	2 oz	?	14	?	278
Pay Day	1.9 oz	?	12	?	250
Pearson's					
Carmel Nip	4	?	3	?	120
Coffee Nip	4	?	3	?	120
Licorice Nip	4	?	3	?	120
Chocolate Parfait	4	?	3	?	120
Peppermint Pattie	1 oz	?	2	?	124
Pillsbury food sticks	4	?	6	?	180
Planters					
peanut bar					
regular	1.6 oz	0	11	2	230
honey roasted	1.6 oz	0	13	2	230
Sweet 'n Crunchy	1.6 oz	0	15	2	250
Old Fashioned peanut candy	1 oz	0	9	1	140
Pom Poms	½ box	?	3	?	100
Power House	1 oz	?	5	?	131
Reese's					
Peanut Butter Cup	1.8 oz	8	17	6	280
peanut butter–flavored chips	¼ c	3	13	11	223
Pieces	1.95 oz	2	11	9	270
Rolo	9 pieces or 1.93 oz	13	12	8	270
Skor	1.4 oz	?	14	?	220
Snickers	2 oz	?	13	?	270
Sno-Caps	1 oz	?	4	?	132
Starbar	1 oz	?	7	?	141
Sugar Babies	1 pkg	?	2	?	180
Sugar Daddy	1	?	1	?	150
Summit	0.76 oz	?	6	?	100
Thousand Dollar	1½ oz	?	8	?	200
Three Musketeers	2.28 oz	?	8	?	280
Twix	1.73 oz	?	6	?	120
Whatchamacallit	1.8 oz	?	15	?	270
Y&S Bites or Twizzlers	1 oz	?	<1	?	100
Zero	2 oz	?	8	?	250

	Portion	Chol (mg)	Total Fat (g)	Satur'd Fat (g)	Total Calor

□ **CANNED MEATS** *See* PROCESSED MEAT & POULTRY PRODUCTS

□ **CEREAL, BREAKFAST** *See* BREAKFAST CEREALS, COLD & HOT

□ **CHEESE & CHEESE FOODS**

Natural Cheese

	Portion	Chol (mg)	Total Fat (g)	Satur'd Fat (g)	Total Calor
bleu	1 oz	21	8	5	100
	1 c, crumbled, not packed	102	39	25	477
brick	1" cube	16	5	3	64
	1 oz	27	8	5	105
Brie	1 oz	28	8	?	95
	4½ oz	128	35	?	427
Camembert	1 oz	20	7	4	85
	3⅓ oz	27	9	6	114
caraway	1 oz	?	8	?	107
cheddar	1 oz	30	9	6	114
	1 c, shredded, not packed	119	37	24	455
Cheshire	1 oz	29	9	?	110
Colby	1" cube	16	6	3	68
	1 oz	27	9	6	112
cottage					
creamed, small curd	4 oz	17	5	3	117
	1 c, not packed	31	9	6	217
fruit added	4 oz	13	4	2	140
	1 c, not packed	25	8	5	279
dry curd	4 oz	8	tr	tr	96
	1 c, not packed	10	tr	tr	123
low-fat					
2%	4 oz	9	2	1	101
	1 c, not packed	19	4	3	203
1%	4 oz	5	1	tr	82
	1 c, not packed	10	2	1	164
cream	1 oz	31	10	6	99
	3 oz	93	30	19	297

	Portion	Chol (mg)	Total Fat (g)	Satur'd Fat (g)	Total Calor
Edam	1 oz	25	8	5	101
	7 oz	177	55	35	706
feta, from sheep's milk	1 oz	25	6	4	75
fontina	1 oz	33	9	5	110
	8 oz	263	71	44	883
gjetost, from goats' &	1 oz	?	8	5	132
cows' milk	8 oz	?	67	43	1,057
Gouda	1 oz	32	8	5	101
	7 oz	226	54	35	705
Gruyère	1 oz	31	9	5	117
	6 oz	187	55	32	702
Limburger	1 oz	26	8	5	93
	8 oz	204	62	38	742
Monterey Jack	1 oz	?	9	?	106
	6 oz	?	51	?	635
mozzarella	1 oz	22	6	4	80
low-moisture	1" cube	16	4	3	56
	1 oz	25	7	4	90
part skim	1" cube	10	3	2	49
	1 oz	15	5	3	79
part skim	1 oz	16	5	3	72
Muenster	1 oz	27	9	5	104
	6 oz	163	51	32	626
Neufchâtel	1 oz	22	7	4	74
	3 oz	65	20	13	221
Parmesan					
grated	1 T	4	2	1	23
	1 oz	22	9	5	129
hard	1 oz	19	7	5	111
	5 oz	96	37	23	557
Port du Salut	1 oz	35	8	5	100
	6 oz	209	48	28	598
provolone	1 oz	20	8	5	100
	6 oz	117	45	29	598
ricotta					
whole milk	½ c	63	16	10	216
part skim milk	½ c	38	10	6	171
Romano, hard	1 oz	29	8	?	110
	5 oz	148	38	?	549
Roquefort, from sheep's	1 oz	26	9	5	105
milk	3 oz	76	26	16	314
Swiss	1" cube	14	4	3	56
	1 oz	20	8	5	107
Tilsit	1 oz	29	7	5	96
	6 oz	173	44	29	578

whey *See* MILK, MILK SUBSTITUTES, & MILK PRODUCTS

	Portion	Chol (mg)	Total Fat (g)	Satur'd Fat (g)	Total Calor

Processed Cheese & Cheese Food

CHEESE FOOD

American					
cold pack	1 oz	18	7	4	94
	8 oz	144	56	35	752
pasteurized process	1 oz	18	7	4	93
	8 oz	145	56	35	745
Swiss, pasteurized process	1 oz	23	7	?	92
	8 oz	186	55	?	734

CHEESE SPREAD

American, pasteurized	1 oz	16	6	4	82
process	5 oz	78	30	19	412

PASTEURIZED PROCESS CHEESE

American	1″ cube	17	5	3	66
	1 oz	27	9	6	106
pimiento	1″ cube	16	5	3	66
	1 oz	27	9	6	106
Swiss	1″ cube	15	4	3	60
	1 oz	24	7	5	95

▪ BRAND NAME

Armour					
cheddar, regular or lower salt	1 oz	30	9	?	110
Colby, regular or lower salt	1 oz	30	9	?	110
Monterey Jack, regular or lower salt	1 oz	30	9	?	110
Bonbel *See* Fromageries Bel, *below*					
Delicia Pasteurized Process Cheese Substitute					
American	1 oz	0	6	?	80
American w/peppers	1 oz	0	6	?	80
Hickory Smoked American	1 oz	0	6	?	80
Featherweight					
cheddar, low-sodium	1 oz	?	9	?	110
Friendship					
cottage cheese					
California style, 4% milk fat	½ c	17	5	?	120
Friendship 'n Fruit low-fat	6 oz	7	1	?	100
regular or lactose-reduced, both 1% milk fat	½ c	5	1	?	90
large curd pot style, 2% milk fat	½ c	9	2	?	100

	Portion	Chol (mg)	Total Fat (g)	Satur'd Fat (g)	Total Calor
cottage cheese *(cont.)*					
w/pineapple, 4% milk fat	½ c	17	4	?	140
cream cheese	1 oz	31	<10	?	103
farmer cheese	½ c	40	12	?	160
natural hoop cheese, ½% milk fat	4 oz	8	<1	?	84
Fromageries Bel					
Babybel	1 oz	22	7	?	91
Bombino	1 oz	27	9	?	103
Bonbel	1 oz	24	8	?	100
cheddar	1 oz	28	9	?	110
Edam	1 oz	26	8	?	100
Gouda	1 oz	28	9	?	110
Mini Babybel	¾ oz	18	6	?	74
Mini Bonbel	¾ oz	18	6	?	74
Mini Gouda	¾ oz	21	6	?	80
Reduced Mini	¾ oz	8	3	?	45
Hoffman's					
CHEESE FOOD					
American	1 oz	?	7	?	100
Chees'n Bacon	1 oz	?	6	?	90
Chees'n Onion	1 oz	?	7	?	100
Chees'n Salami	1 oz	?	6	?	90
Hot Pepper w/jalapeño peppers	1 oz	?	7	?	90
Swisson Rye w/caraway	1 oz	?	7	?	90
PASTEURIZED PROCESS CHEESE					
American	1 oz	?	9	?	110
cheddar					
Smokey Sharp	1 oz	?	9	?	110
Super Sharp	1 oz	?	8	?	110
Smokey Swiss'n Cheddar	1 oz	?	8	?	110
Land O'Lakes					
CULTURED CHEESE					
cottage cheese	4 oz	15	5	3	120
cottage cheese, 2% milk fat	4 oz	10	2	1	100
NATURAL CHEESE					
brick	1 oz	25	8	5	110
cheddar	1 oz	30	9	6	110
Colby	1 oz	25	9	6	110
Edam	1 oz	25	8	5	100
Gouda	1 oz	30	8	5	100
Monterey Jack	1 oz	20	9	5	110
mozzarella, low-moisture, part skim	1 oz	15	5	3	80
Muenster	1 oz	25	9	5	100
provolone	1 oz	20	8	5	100

	Portion	Chol (mg)	Total Fat (g)	Satur'd Fat (g)	Total Calor
Swiss	1 oz	25	8	5	110
PROCESSED CHEESE & CHEESE FOOD					
American	1 oz	25	9	6	110
Golden Velvet cheese spread	1 oz	15	6	4	80
jalapeño cheese food	1 oz	20	7	4	90
onion cheese food	1 oz	15	7	4	90
pepperoni cheese food	1 oz	20	7	4	90
Laughing Cow					
average values of cheese spreads	1 oz	18	6	?	78
May-Bud					
Edam	1 oz	?	8	?	100
farmers, semisoft, part skim	1 oz	?	7	?	90
Gouda	1 oz	?	8	?	100
Monterey Jack	1 oz	?	9	?	110
Nabisco Easy Cheese					
pasteurized process cheese spread, all flavors	1 oz	?	6	?	80
Wispride Cold Pack Cheese Food					
port wine	1 oz	25	7	?	100
sharp cheddar	1 oz	25	7	?	100

❑ **CHICKEN** *See* POULTRY, FRESH & PROCESSED

❑ **CHUTNEYS** *See* PICKLES, OLIVES, RELISHES, & CHUTNEYS

❑ **COATINGS, SEASONED** *See* BREADCRUMBS, CROUTONS, STUFFINGS, & SEASONED COATINGS

❑ **CONDIMENTS** *See* SAUCES, GRAVIES, & CONDIMENTS

	Portion	Chol (mg)	Total Fat (g)	Satur'd Fat (g)	Total Calor

❑ COOKIES, BARS, & BROWNIES

	Portion	Chol (mg)	Total Fat (g)	Satur'd Fat (g)	Total Calor
animal cookies	15	?	3	?	120
arrowroot cookies	2	?	2	?	47
brownies					
butterscotch	1 oz	?	5	?	115
chocolate, from mix	1.1 oz	?	5	?	130
chocolate, w/nuts					
commercial, frosted	0.9 oz	14	4	2	100
homemade, w/vegetable oil	0.7 oz	18	6	1	95
cherry coolers	2	?	2	?	58
chocolate chip cookies					
commercial	4 (2¼" diam)	5	9	3	180
from refrigerator dough	4 (2¼" diam)	22	11	4	225
homemade, w/vegetable shortening	4 (2⅓" diam)	18	11	4	185
w/coconut	1	?	4	?	82
chocolate cookies	1	?	3	?	93
chocolate sandwich cookies	1	?	2	?	49
chocolate snaps	4	?	2	?	53
coconut bars	1	?	5	?	109
fig bars	4 = 2 oz	27	4	1	210
gingersnaps					
commercial	3 small	?	1	?	50
homemade	1	?	2	?	34
golden fruit cookies	1	?	1	?	63
graham crackers	2	0	1	tr	60
chocolate-covered	1	?	3	?	62
granola bars	1	?	4	?	109
lemon coolers	2	?	2	?	57
macaroons	1	?	3	?	67
molasses cookies	1	?	3	?	71
oatmeal cookies					
commercial	1	?	3	?	80
from mix	2	?	6	?	130
homemade	1	?	3	?	62
oatmeal chocolate chip cookies	1	?	3	?	57
oatmeal raisin cookies					
from refrigerator dough	1	?	3	?	61
homemade	4 (2⅝" diam)	2	10	3	245
peanut butter bars	1	?	10	?	198
peanut butter cookies					
from refrigerator dough	1	?	3	?	50
homemade	4 = 1.7 oz	28	14	4	245
peanut cookies	1	?	2	?	57

	Portion	Chol (mg)	Total Fat (g)	Satur'd Fat (g)	Total Calor
sandwich-type cookies, chocolate or vanilla	4 = 1.4 oz	0	8	2	195
shortbread cookies					
commercial	4 small	27	8	3	155
homemade, w/margarine	2 large	0	8	1	145
social tea cookies	2	?	1	?	43
sugar cookies					
from mix	2	?	5	?	120
from refrigerator dough	4 = 1.7 oz	29	12	2	235
homemade	1	?	3	?	89
sugar wafers	2	?	2	?	53
vanilla cream sandwich cookies	1	?	3	?	69
vanilla wafers	10 = 1.4 oz	25	7	2	185
Vienna dream bars, from mix	1	?	5	?	90
Vienna finger sandwich cookies	1	?	3	?	72

▪ BRAND NAME

Famous Amos

	Portion	Chol (mg)	Total Fat (g)	Satur'd Fat (g)	Total Calor
chocolate chip, no nuts, extra chips	1 oz	?	8	?	147
chocolate chip w/macadamia nuts	1 oz	?	9	?	152
chocolate chip w/pecans	1 oz	?	8	?	151
oatmeal w/cinnamon & raisins	1 oz	?	6	?	133

Health Valley

	Portion	Chol (mg)	Total Fat (g)	Satur'd Fat (g)	Total Calor
Animal Snaps, cinnamon or vanilla	6	0	1	?	15
fruit bars, apple, date, or raisin	2	0	4	?	180
Fruit Jumbos					
almonds & dates or raisins & nuts	1	0	3	?	85
oat bran	1	0	3	?	80
tropical fruit	1	0	3	?	85
graham crackers					
amaranth	3	0	1	?	50
oat bran	3	0	2	?	54
Jumbos					
amaranth	1	0	2	?	60
cinnamon	1	0	2	?	70
oatmeal	1	0	2	?	60
peanut butter	1	0	2	?	70
tofu cookies	4	0	3	?	52
wheat-free cookies	4	0	3	?	52

	Portion	Chol (mg)	Total Fat (g)	Satur'd Fat (g)	Total Calor
Hershey New Trail Granola Snack Bars					
chocolate chip	1	?	9	?	190
chocolate-covered cocoa creme	1	?	12	?	200
chocolate-covered honey graham	1	?	12	?	200
chocolate-covered peanut butter	1	?	11	?	200
peanut butter	1	?	9	?	190
peanut butter & chocolate chip	1	?	9	?	180
Kellogg's Rice Krispies Bars					
chocolate chip	1	?	4	?	120
Cocoa Krispies chocolate chip	1	?	4	?	120
raisin	1	?	2	?	120
Nabisco					
Almost Home Family-Style cookies					
fudge chocolate chip cookies	2	?	5	?	130
fudge & nut brownies	1	?	7	?	160
fudge & vanilla creme sandwiches	1	?	6	?	140
iced Dutch apple fruit sticks	1	?	1	?	70
oatmeal raisin cookies	2	?	5	?	130
peanut butter chocolate chip cookies	2	?	6	?	140
Real chocolate chip cookies	2	?	5	?	130
Old Fashioned sugar cookies	2	?	5	?	130
Apple Newtons	1	?	2	?	110
Barnum's Animals (animal crackers)	11	?	4	?	130
Bugs Bunny graham cookies	9	?	4	?	120
Cameo creme sandwiches	2	?	5	?	140
Chewy Chips Ahoy!	2	?	6	?	130
Chips 'n More	2	?	7	?	150
chocolate grahams	3	?	7	?	150
chocolate snaps	7	?	4	?	130
Cinnamon Treats	2	?	1	?	60
Cookies 'n Fudge	3	?	8	?	150
devil's food cakes	1	?	1	?	110
Famous chocolate wafers	5	?	4	?	130
Giggles vanilla sandwich cookies	2	?	6	?	140

	Portion	Chol (mg)	Total Fat (g)	Satur'd Fat (g)	Total Calor
graham or Honey Maid graham crackers	2	?	1	?	60
imported Danish cookies	5	?	8	?	150
I Screams n' You Screams Double Dip chocolate creme sandwiches	2	?	7	?	150
Lorna Doone shortbread	4	?	7	?	140
Mallomars	2	?	6	?	130
National arrowroot biscuits	6	?	4	?	130
Old Fashion ginger snaps	4	?	3	?	120
Oreo chocolate sandwich cookies	3	?	6	?	140
Oreo mint creme chocolate sandwich cookies	2	?	6	?	150
Pantry molasses cookies	2	?	4	?	130
pecan shortbread cookies	2	?	9	?	150
Pinwheels	1	?	5	?	130
Social Tea biscuits	6	?	4	?	130

Pepperidge Farm
ASSORTMENT COOKIES

	Portion	Chol (mg)	Total Fat (g)	Satur'd Fat (g)	Total Calor
Champagne	2	?	6	?	110
Original Pirouettes	2	?	6	?	110
Seville	2	?	5	?	100

DISTINCTIVE COOKIES

	Portion	Chol (mg)	Total Fat (g)	Satur'd Fat (g)	Total Calor
Bordeaux	3	?	5	?	110
Brussels	3	?	9	?	170
Chessmen	3	?	6	?	130
Geneva	3	?	11	?	190
Lido	2	?	11	?	180
Milano	3	?	7	?	130
Nassau	2	?	10	?	170
Orleans	3	?	5	?	100

FRUIT COOKIES

	Portion	Chol (mg)	Total Fat (g)	Satur'd Fat (g)	Total Calor
apricot-raspberry	3	?	6	?	150

KITCHEN HEARTH COOKIES

	Portion	Chol (mg)	Total Fat (g)	Satur'd Fat (g)	Total Calor
date nut granola	3	?	8	?	170
raisin bran	3	?	8	?	160

OLD FASHIONED COOKIES

	Portion	Chol (mg)	Total Fat (g)	Satur'd Fat (g)	Total Calor
brownie chocolate nut	3	?	10	?	170
chocolate chip	3	?	7	?	150
chocolate chocolate chip	3	?	8	?	160
Gingerman	3	?	4	?	100
hazelnut	3	?	8	?	170
Irish oatmeal	3	?	6	?	150
Lemon Nut Crunch	3	?	10	?	180
Molasses Crisps	3	?	4	?	100

	Portion	Chol (mg)	Total Fat (g)	Satur'd Fat (g)	Total Calor
oatmeal raisin	3	?	7	?	170
shortbread	3	?	7	?	130
sugar	3	?	7	?	150
SPECIAL COLLECTION COOKIES					
Almond Supreme	2	?	10	?	140
Chocolate Chunk Pecan	2	?	7	?	130
milk chocolate macadamia	2	?	8	?	140
Pillsbury					
all cookies	3	?	≤10	?	varies
Quaker Oats					
CHEWY GRANOLA BARS					
chocolate chip	1	?	5	?	129
chocolate, graham, & marshmallow	1	?	4	?	126
chunky nut & raisin	1	?	6	?	133
honey & oats	1	?	4	?	125
peanut butter	1	?	5	?	130
raisin & cinnamon	1	?	5	?	130
GRANOLA DIPPS BARS					
chocolate chip	1	?	6	?	138
honey & oats	1	?	6	?	137
peanut butter	1	?	7	?	141
raisin & almond	1	?	6	?	139
Rokeach					
graham crackers	8	?	3	?	120
Sunshine					
animal crackers	14	0	3	?	120
butter-flavored cookies	4	5	5	?	120
Chip-A-Roos	2	0	7	?	130
Chips'n Middles	2	0	6	?	140
chocolate fudge sandwiches	2	0	7	?	150
cinnamon graham crackers	4, after breaking	0	3	?	70
Country Style oatmeal cookies	2	0	5	?	110
fig bars	2	0	2	?	90
ginger snaps	5	0	3	?	100
Golden Fruit raisin biscuits	2, after breaking	0	3	?	150
honey graham crackers	4, after breaking	0	2	?	60
Hydrox	3	0	7	?	160
Mallopuffs	2	0	4	?	140
sugar wafers	3	0	6	?	130
vanilla wafers	6	5	6	?	130
Vienna fingers	2	0	6	?	140

	Portion	Chol (mg)	Total Fat (g)	Satur'd Fat (g)	Total Calor

❏ CORNMEAL *See* FLOURS & CORNMEALS

❏ CRACKERS
See also SNACKS

	Portion	Chol (mg)	Total Fat (g)	Satur'd Fat (g)	Total Calor
bread sticks *See* BREADS, ROLLS, BISCUITS, & MUFFINS					
cheese, plain	10 (1" square)	6	3	1	50
cheese & peanut butter sandwich	1	1	2	tr	40
graham *See* COOKIES, BARS, & BROWNIES					
matzo	1	?	tr	?	117
melba toast, plain	1	0	tr	tr	20
oyster	33	?	3	?	120
rice wafers	3	?	0	?	31
rusk	1	?	1	?	42
rye crisp	2 triple crackers	?	tr	?	50
rye wafers, whole-grain	2 = ½ oz	0	1	tr	55
saltines	4	4	1	1	50
snack-type crackers, standard, round	1	0	1	tr	15
soda, unsalted tops	10	?	3	?	120
taco shells *See* BREADS, ROLLS, BISCUITS, & MUFFINS					
tortillas *See* BREADS, ROLLS, BISCUITS, & MUFFINS					
wheat, thin	4	0	1	1	35
whole-wheat wafers	2	0	2	1	35
zwieback *See* INFANT & TODDLER FOODS					

▪ BRAND NAME

	Portion	Chol (mg)	Total Fat (g)	Satur'd Fat (g)	Total Calor
Cracottes					
regular or salt-free	1	?	tr	tr	12
whole-wheat	1	?	tr	tr	13
Featherweight					
crackers	2	?	1	?	30
wafers, bran or wheat	4	?	1	?	50
Health Valley					
Cheese Wheels	12	3	7	?	140
French onion, regular or no salt	13	0	6	?	130
herb, regular or no salt	13	0	6	?	130
honey graham	13	0	6	?	130

	Portion	Chol (mg)	Total Fat (g)	Satur'd Fat (g)	Total Calor
sesame, regular or no salt	13	0	6	?	130
7-Grain Vegetable					
regular	1 oz	0	6	?	130
no salt	1 oz	0	5	?	120
stoned-wheat, regular or no salt	13	0	6	?	130
Nabisco					
Bacon-Flavored Thins	7	?	4	?	70
Better Blue Cheese	10	?	4	?	70
Better Cheddars	11	?	4	?	70
Better Cheddars 'n' Bacon	10	?	4	?	70
Better Nachos	9	?	4	?	70
Better Swiss Cheese	10	?	4	?	70
cheese peanut butter sandwiches	2	?	3	?	70
Cheese Tid-Bits	16	?	4	?	70
Cheese Wheat Thins	9	?	3	?	70
Chicken in a Biskit	7	?	4	?	70
Crown Pilot	1	?	1	?	60
Dandy Soup & Oyster	20	?	1	?	60
Dip in a Chip Cheese 'n Chive	8	?	4	?	70
Escort	3	?	4	?	80
graham or Honey Maid graham crackers *See* COOKIES, BARS, & BROWNIES					
Great Crisps! *See* SNACKS					
Holland Rusk	1	?	1	?	60
Meal Mates	3	?	3	?	70
Nips *See* SNACKS					
Nutty Wheat Thins	7	?	5	?	80
Oysterettes	18	?	1	?	60
Premium saltines, regular or low-salt	5	?	2	?	60
Ritz					
regular or low-salt	4	?	4	?	70
cheese	5	?	3	?	70
Royal Lunch Milk	1	?	2	?	60
Sea Rounds	1	?	2	?	60
Sociables	6	?	3	?	70
Toasted Peanut Butter Sandwiches	2	?	4	?	70
Triscuits, regular or low-salt	3	?	2	?	60
Twigs, sesame or cheese	5	?	4	?	70
Uneeda Biscuit, unsalted tops	3	?	2	?	60
Vegetable Thins	7	?	4	?	70
Waverly	4	?	3	?	70
Wheatsworth	5	?	3	?	70
Wheat Thins, regular or low-salt	8	?	3	?	70

	Portion	Chol (mg)	Total Fat (g)	Satur'd Fat (g)	Total Calor
Pepperidge Farm					
butter-flavored thin crackers	4	?	3	?	80
English water biscuits	4	?	1	?	70
Hearty wheat crackers	4	?	4	?	100
sesame crackers	4	?	3	?	80
Snack Sticks *See* SNACKS					
Tiny Goldfish *See* SNACKS					
Pillsbury					
bread sticks *See* BREADS, ROLLS, BISCUITS, & MUFFINS					
Quaker Oats					
rice cakes, lightly salted: plain, multigrain, or sesame	1	0	tr	?	35
Rokeach					
saltines	10	?	3	?	120
snack crackers	9	?	5	?	130
Sunshine					
American Heritage					
cheddar	5	5	4	?	80
sesame	4	0	4	?	70
Cheez-It	12	0	4	?	70
Hi Ho	4	0	5	?	80
Krispy saltines	5	0	1	?	60
oyster & soup	16	0	2	?	60
wheat wafers	8	0	4	?	80

❑ CREAM & CREAM SUBSTITUTES
See MILK, MILK SUBSTITUTES, & MILK PRODUCTS

❑ CROUTONS *See* BREADCRUMBS, CROUTONS, STUFFINGS, & SEASONED COATINGS

❑ CUSTARDS *See* DESSERTS: CUSTARDS, GELATINS, PUDDINGS, & PIE FILLINGS

❑ DELI MEATS *See* PROCESSED MEAT & POULTRY PRODUCTS

	Portion	Chol (mg)	Total Fat (g)	Satur'd Fat (g)	Total Calor

❑ **DESSERTS: CAKES, PASTRIES, & PIES**

Cake & Coffee Cake

	Portion	Chol (mg)	Total Fat (g)	Satur'd Fat (g)	Total Calor
angel food					
from mix	whole (9¾″ diam tube)	0	2	tr	1,510
	¹⁄₁₂ cake	0	tr	tr	125
homemade	2.1 oz	?	tr	?	161
applesauce spice, from mix	¹⁄₁₂ cake	?	11	?	250
banana, from mix	¹⁄₁₂ cake	?	11	?	260
w/buttercream icing	1.8 oz	?	7	?	181
Boston cream pie	3.9 oz	?	10	?	332
butter brickle, from mix	¹⁄₁₂ cake	?	11	?	260
butter pecan, from mix	⅛ cake	?	15	?	310
	¹⁄₁₂ cake	?	11	?	250
caramel, from mix	1.6 oz	?	8	?	173
w/caramel icing	1.9 oz	?	8	?	208
carrot					
from mix	¹⁄₁₂ cake	?	11	?	250
homemade, w/cream cheese icing	whole (10″ diam tube)	1,183	328	66	6,175
	¹⁄₁₆ cake	74	21	4	385
cheesecake					
commercial	whole (9″ diam)	2,053	213	120	3,350
	¹⁄₁₂ cake	170	18	10	280
from mix	⅛ cake	30	14	9	300
cherry chip, from mix	¹⁄₁₂ cake	?	3	?	180
chocolate	¹⁄₁₂ cake	?	11	?	250
w/icing, from mix	1.3 oz cupcake	?	5	?	129
chocolate chip, from mix	¹⁄₁₂ cake	?	4	?	190
chocolate fudge bundt ring, from mix	¹⁄₁₆ cake	?	12	?	270
chocolate fudge w/vanilla icing, from mix	⅙ cake	?	10	?	280
chocolate macaroon bundt ring, from mix	¹⁄₁₆ cake	?	11	?	250
chocolate mint, from mix	¹⁄₁₂ cake	?	12	?	250
chocolate pudding, from mix	⅙ cake	?	5	?	230
cinnamon streusel, from mix	⅛ cake	?	8	?	250

	Portion	Chol (mg)	Total Fat (g)	Satur'd Fat (g)	Total Calor
coffee cake, crumb, from mix	whole (15.1 oz)	279	41	12	1,385
	⅙ cake	47	7	2	230
cottage pudding, home-made	1.8 oz	?	6	?	172
w/chocolate sauce	2½ oz	?	6	?	223
w/fruit sauce	2½ oz	?	6	?	204
devil's food, w/chocolate icing					
from mix, made w/margarine	whole, 2-layer (8" or 9" diam)	598	136	56	3,755
	1/16 cake	37	8	4	235
	1.2 oz cupcake	19	4	2	120
homemade	2.1 oz	?	11	?	233
fruitcake					
dark, homemade	3 lbs	640	228	48	5,185
	1½ oz	20	7	2	165
light	1.4 oz	?	7	?	156
German chocolate, from mix	1/12 cake	?	11	?	260
gingerbread, from mix	whole (8" square)	6	39	10	1,575
	⅑ cake	1	4	1	175
lemon, from mix	1/12 cake	?	11	?	260
lemon bundt ring, from mix	1/16 cake	?	10	?	270
lemon chiffon, from mix	1/12 cake	?	4	?	190
lemon pudding, from mix	⅙ cake	?	5	?	230
marble, from mix	1/12 cake	?	11	?	270
w/white icing	1.8 oz	?	4	?	165
marble streusel, w/icing, from mix	2.3 oz	?	10	?	224
orange					
from mix	1/12 cake	?	11	?	260
homemade, w/icing	1.8 oz	?	7	?	183
pineapple upside-down					
from mix	⅑ cake	?	10	?	270
homemade	2.6 oz	?	9	?	236
plum pudding, canned	3.6 oz	?	1	?	270
pound					
commercial	1.1 lb loaf	1,100	94	52	1,935
	1 oz	64	5	3	110
from mix	1/12 cake	?	9	?	200
homemade	1.1 lb loaf	555	94	21	2,025
	1 oz	32	5	1	120

	Portion	Chol (mg)	Total Fat (g)	Satur'd Fat (g)	Total Calor
sheet, plain, homemade, w/vegetable oil					
unfrosted	whole (9" square)	552	108	30	2,830
	⅑ cake	61	12	3	315
w/uncooked white icing	whole (9" square)	636	129	42	4,020
	⅑ cake	70	14	5	445
shortcake	0.9 oz	?	2	?	86
w/blackberries	5.2 oz	?	8	?	347
w/peaches	5.3 oz	?	6	?	266
w/raspberries	5.6 oz	?	7	?	290
w/strawberries	6.2 oz	?	9	?	344
snack cake, small, commercial					
devil's food w/cream filling	1 oz	15	4	2	105
sponge w/cream filling	1½ oz	7	5	2	155
sour cream, from mix	⅛ cake	?	12	?	270
chocolate	1/12 cake	?	11	?	260
white	1/12 cake	?	3	?	180
spice, from mix	1.8 oz	?	6	?	175
w/vanilla icing	1.8 oz	?	5	?	176
sponge, homemade	2.3 oz	?	3	?	188
w/strawberries & whipped cream	5.4 oz	?	8	?	328
strawberry, from mix	1/12 cake	?	11	?	260
streusel swirl, from mix	1/16 cake	?	11	?	260
white					
from mix	2½ oz	?	10	?	219
homemade	2.7 oz	?	12	?	285
white, w/chocolate icing, homemade	2.7 oz	?	12	?	298
white, w/white icing, commercial	whole, 2-layer (8" or 9" diam)	46	148	33	4,170
	1/16 cake	3	9	2	260
yellow, homemade	2.6 oz	?	12	?	283
yellow, w/chocolate icing					
commercial	whole, 2-layer (8" or 9" diam)	609	175	92	3,895
	1/16 cake	38	11	6	245
from mix	whole, 2-layer (8" or 9" diam)	576	125	48	3,735
	1/16 cake	36	8	3	235
homemade	2.6 oz	?	12	?	292

	Portion	Chol (mg)	Total Fat (g)	Satur'd Fat (g)	Total Calor
yellow cupcake					
w/chocolate icing	1.4 oz	?	5	?	155
w/vanilla icing	1.4 oz	?	6	?	160

Cake Icing

caramel	1.4 oz	?	5	?	140
chocolate	1.4 oz	?	6	?	148
chocolate, double dark	1.3 oz	?	4	?	150
chocolate fudge	1.4 oz	?	4	?	150
coconut	1.4 oz	?	3	?	140
coconut almond	1.2 oz	?	10	?	170
coconut pecan	1.2 oz	?	8	?	150
lemon	1.2 oz	?	5	?	140
milk chocolate	1.1 oz	?	5	?	150
strawberry	1.1 oz	?	5	?	140
vanilla	1.3 oz	?	5	?	150
white, fluffy	0.6 oz	?	0	?	70

Danish, Doughnuts, Sweet Rolls, & Toaster Pastries

danish pastry					
plain, w/out fruit or nuts	12 oz ring	292	71	29	1,305
	1 (4¼" diam)	49	12	4	220
	1 oz	24	6	2	110
cinnamon raisin, from refrigerator dough	2.7 oz	?	11	?	270
fruit	1 round	56	13	4	235
doughnut					
cake type, plain	1.8 oz	20	12	3	210
yeast-leavened, glazed	2.1 oz	21	13	5	235
sweet roll	1	?	7	?	154
cinnamon w/icing, from refrigerator dough	2	?	8	?	230
toaster pastries	1	0	6	2	210

Fruit Bettys, Cobblers, Crisps, & Turnovers

apple brown Betty	½ c	?	5	?	211
apple crisp	½ c	?	8	?	302
apple dumpling	1	?	17	?	280
cherry crisp	½ c	?	tr	?	226
peach cobbler	⅓ c	?	6	?	160
peach crisp	½ c	?	9	?	249
turnover, from mix, apple, blueberry, or cherry	1	?	8	?	173

	Portion	Chol (mg)	Total Fat (g)	Satur'd Fat (g)	Total Calor
Pastry					
cream puff, w/custard filling	3.7 oz	?	15	?	245
éclair					
w/chocolate icing & custard filling	3.9 oz	?	15	?	316
frozen	2 oz	?	10	?	205
w/chocolate icing & whipped cream filling	3.7 oz	?	26	?	296
lady finger, w/whipped cream filling	4 oz	?	17	?	326
pastry shells & pie crusts *See* BAKING INGREDIENTS					
Pie					
apple, w/vegetable shortening crust	whole (9″ diam)	0	105	27	2,420
	⅙ pie	0	18	5	405
banana custard, homemade	5.6 oz	?	15	?	353
blackberry, homemade	5.6 oz	?	18	?	389
blueberry, w/vegetable shortening crust	whole (9″ diam)	0	102	26	2,285
	⅙ pie	0	17	4	380
butterscotch, homemade	5.6 oz	?	18	?	427
cherry, w/vegetable shortening crust	whole (9″ diam)	0	107	28	2,465
	⅙ pie	0	18	5	410
chocolate chiffon, homemade	2.8 oz	?	12	?	262
chocolate cream, homemade	4 oz	?	17	?	301
coconut custard, homemade	5½ oz	?	19	?	365
cream, w/vegetable shortening crust	whole (9″ diam)	46	139	90	2,710
	⅙ pie	8	23	15	455
custard, w/vegetable shortening crust	whole (9″ diam)	1,010	101	34	1,985
	⅙ pie	169	17	6	330
fried					
apple	3 oz	14	14	6	255
cherry	3 oz	13	14	6	250
lemon chiffon, homemade	3.8 oz	?	10	?	288
lemon meringue, w/vegetable shortening crust	whole (9″ diam)	857	86	26	2,140
	⅙ pie	143	14	4	355
mincemeat, homemade	5.6 oz	?	18	?	434
peach, w/vegetable shortening crust	whole (9″ diam)	0	101	25	2,410
	⅙ pie	0	17	4	405

	Portion	Chol (mg)	Total Fat (g)	Satur'd Fat (g)	Total Calor
pecan, w/vegetable shortening crust	whole (9″ diam)	569	189	28	3,450
	⅙ pie	95	32	5	575
pineapple cheese, homemade	5.6 oz	?	10	?	270
pumpkin, w/vegetable shortening crust	whole (9″ diam)	655	102	38	1,920
	⅙ pie	109	17	6	320
raisin, homemade	4.2 oz	?	13	?	325
rhubarb, homemade	5.6 oz	?	17	?	405
shoofly, homemade	3.9 oz	?	16	?	441
strawberry, homemade	4 oz	?	9	?	228
sweet potato, homemade	5.6 oz	?	18	?	342

Pie Fillings *See* DESSERTS: CUSTARDS, GELATINS, PUDDINGS, & PIE FILLINGS

▪ BRAND NAME

Dromedary
date nut roll	½″ slice	?	2	?	80

Kellogg's
FROSTED POP-TARTS
blueberry	1	?	5	?	200
brown sugar cinnamon	1	?	7	?	210
chocolate fudge	1	?	4	?	200
Dutch apple	1	?	6	?	210
peanut butter & jelly	1	?	9	?	220

POP-TARTS
blueberry	1	?	5	?	210
brown sugar cinnamon	1	?	8	?	210

Nabisco
Frosted Toastettes or Toastettes, all flavors	1	?	5	?	200

Pepperidge Farm Frozen Cakes & Pastries
FRUIT SQUARES
apple	1	?	12	?	220
blueberry	1	?	11	?	220
cherry	1	?	12	?	230

LAYER CAKES
coconut	1⅝ oz	?	8	?	180
devil's food	1⅝ oz	?	8	?	170
German chocolate	1⅝ oz	?	10	?	180
golden	1⅝ oz	?	9	?	180

	Portion	Chol (mg)	Total Fat (g)	Satur'd Fat (g)	Total Calor
vanilla	1⅝ oz	?	8	?	170

OLD FASHIONED CAKES

butter pound	1 oz	?	6	?	120
carrot w/cream cheese icing	1⅜ oz	?	7	?	130

PUFF PASTRY

apple dumplings	3 oz	?	13	?	260
apple strudel	3 oz	?	10	?	240
patty shells	1	?	15	?	210
puff pastry sheets	¼ sheet	?	17	?	260
turnovers					
apple	1	?	17	?	300
blueberry	1	?	19	?	310
cherry	1	?	19	?	310
peach	1	?	18	?	310
raspberry	1	?	17	?	310

SUPREME CAKES

Boston cream	2⅞ oz	?	14	?	290
chocolate	2⅞ oz	?	16	?	300
Grand Marnier	1½ oz	?	18	?	160
lemon coconut	3 oz	?	13	?	280
raspberry mocha	3⅛ oz	?	14	?	310
strawberry cream	2 oz	?	7	?	190

Pillsbury
SWEET ROLLS

Best apple danish w/icing	1	?	11	?	240
Best quick cinnamon rolls w/icing	1	?	9	?	210
cinnamon raisin danish w/ icing	2	?	14	?	290
cinnamon w/icing	2	?	9	?	230

TURNOVERS

all flavors	1	?	8	?	170

Rich's

Bavarian cream puffs	1	35	8	?	146
chocolate éclairs	2 oz	35	10	?	205

Sara Lee
ALL BUTTER COFFEE CAKES

butter streusel	⅛ cake	?	7	?	160
cheese	⅛ cake	?	12	?	210
pecan	⅛ cake	?	8	?	160

ALL BUTTER POUND CAKES

Original	⅒ cake	?	7	?	130
Family Size	1/15 cake	?	7	?	130

	Portion	Chol (mg)	Total Fat (g)	Satur'd Fat (g)	Total Calor
chocolate chip	⅒ cake	?	5	?	130
walnut raisin	⅒ cake	?	5	?	140
ELEGANT ENDINGS					
Classic	⅙ pkg	?	22	?	350
INDIVIDUAL DANISH					
apple	1	?	6	?	120
cheese	1	?	8	?	130
cinnamon raisin	1	?	8	?	150
raspberry	1	?	6	?	130
LE PASTRIE CROISSANTS					
apple	1	?	11	?	260
chocolate	1	?	18	?	320
cinnamon-nut-raisin	1	?	17	?	350
strawberry	1	?	11	?	270
LIGHT CLASSICS					
French cheesecake					
plain	⅒ pkg	?	13	?	200
strawberry	⅒ pkg	?	11	?	200
mousse cake					
chocolate	⅒ pkg	?	14	?	200
strawberry	⅒ pkg	?	11	?	180
SINGLE-LAYER ICED CAKES					
banana	⅛ cake	?	6	?	170
carrot	⅛ cake	?	13	?	260
TWO-LAYER CAKES					
Black Forest	⅛ cake	?	8	?	190
strawberry shortcake	⅛ cake	?	8	?	190

▢ DESSERTS: CUSTARDS, GELATINS, PUDDINGS, & PIE FILLINGS

Custard

	Portion	Chol (mg)	Total Fat (g)	Satur'd Fat (g)	Total Calor
plain					
baked, homemade	½ c	?	7	?	153
boiled, homemade	½ c	?	7	?	164
from mix	½ c	80	5	3	161
banana	½ c	?	5	?	143
chocolate	½ c	?	4	?	142
coconut	½ c	?	4	?	144
lemon	½ c	?	5	?	143
vanilla	½ c	?	5	?	143

	Portion	Chol (mg)	Total Fat (g)	Satur'd Fat (g)	Total Calor
Gelatin					
dry	1 envelope	0	tr	tr	25
made w/water, all flavors	½ c	0	tr	tr	81
Bavarian (w/whipped cream)					
chocolate	1 serving	?	23	?	331
strawberry	1 serving	?	18	?	227
Pie Filling					
pumpkin pie mix, canned	½ c	0	tr	tr	141
Pudding					
butterscotch, homemade	½ c	?	5	?	207
chocolate					
canned	5 oz	1	11	10	205
from mix, prepared w/ whole milk					
regular	½ c	15	4	2	150
instant	½ c	14	4	2	155
homemade	½ c	?	7	?	219
Indian, baked, homemade	⅔ c	?	6	?	161
lemon snow, homemade	½ c	?	tr	?	114
rice, from mix, prepared w/whole milk	½ c	15	4	2	155
rice w/raisins, homemade	¾ c	?	5	?	212
tapioca					
canned	5 oz	tr	5	5	160
from mix, prepared w/ whole milk	½ c	15	4	2	145
homemade	½ c	?	5	?	133
vanilla					
canned	5 oz	1	10	10	220
from mix, prepared w/ whole milk					
regular	½ c	15	4	2	145
instant	½ c	15	4	2	150
homemade	½ c	?	5	?	152
Rennin Dessert					
plain, homemade	½ c	?	4	?	113
chocolate, from mix					
prepared w/whole milk	½ c	?	18	?	127
prepared w/skim milk	½ c	?	1	?	95
fruit vanilla, from mix					
prepared w/whole milk	½ c	?	5	?	140
prepared w/skim milk	½ c	?	tr	?	88

	Portion	Chol (mg)	Total Fat (g)	Satur'd Fat (g)	Total Calor

- **BRAND NAME**

D-Zerta

gelatin, low-cal	½ c	0	0	0	8
pudding, reduced-calorie, prepared w/skim milk					
chocolate	½ c	0	0	0	60
vanilla	½ c	0	0	0	70

Featherweight

custard, lemon or vanilla	½ c	?	0	0	40
gelatin, low-sodium, low-cal, all flavors	½ c	?	0	0	10
mousse, low-cal, chocolate	½ c	?	3	?	85
pudding: butterscotch, chocolate, or vanilla	½ c	?	0	?	12

Jell-O

AMERICANA DESSERTS, PREPARED W/WHOLE MILK

golden egg custard	½ c	80	5	?	160
rice pudding	½ c	15	4	?	170
tapioca pudding					
chocolate	½ c	15	5	?	170
vanilla	½ c	15	4	?	160

GELATIN

average values, all flavors	½ c	0	0	0	80

PUDDING & PIE FILLING

Regular, Prepared w/Whole Milk

butterscotch	½ c	15	4	?	170
chocolate	½ c	15	4	?	160
vanilla	½ c	15	4	?	160

Instant, Prepared w/Whole Milk

banana cream	½ c	15	4	?	160
butterscotch	½ c	15	4	?	160
chocolate	½ c	15	4	?	180
lemon	½ c	15	4	?	170
vanilla	½ c	15	4	?	170

Sugar-free, Prepared w/2% Low-Fat Milk

chocolate	½ c	10	3	?	90
vanilla	½ c	10	2	?	80

Sugar-free Instant, Prepared w/2% Low-Fat Milk

banana	½ c	10	2	?	90
butterscotch	½ c	10	2	?	90

	Portion	Chol (mg)	Total Fat (g)	Satur'd Fat (g)	Total Calor
chocolate	½ c	10	3	?	100
vanilla	½ c	10	2	?	90

RICH & DELICIOUS MOUSSE, PREPARED W/WHOLE MILK

chocolate or chocolate fudge	½ c	10	6	?	150

Rich's Puddings

butterscotch	3 oz	0	6	?	133
chocolate	3 oz	0	7	?	141
vanilla	3 oz	0	6	?	129

Royal
GELATIN

all flavors					
regular	½ c	?	0	?	80
sugar-free	½ c	?	0	?	6

PUDDING & PIE FILLING
Cooked

banana cream, prepared	½ c	?	4	?	160
butterscotch, prepared	½ c	?	4	?	160
chocolate					
dry	0.9 oz	?	1	?	120
prepared	½ c	?	4	?	180
custard, prepared	½ c	?	5	?	150
Dark 'n Sweet, prepared	½ c	?	4	?	180
flan w/caramel sauce, prepared	½ c	?	5	?	150
key lime, prepared	½ c	?	3	?	160
lemon					
dry	½ oz	?	0	?	50
prepared	½ c	?	3	?	160
vanilla					
dry	0.7 oz	?	1	?	80
prepared	½ c	?	4	?	160

Instant

banana cream, prepared	½ c	?	5	?	180
butterscotch, prepared	½ c	?	5	?	180
chocolate					
dry	1 oz	?	1	?	120
prepared	½ c	?	4	?	190
Dark 'n Sweet, prepared	½ c	?	4	?	190
lemon					
dry	0.8 oz	?	1	?	110
prepared	½ c	?	5	?	180
pistachio nut, prepared	½ c	?	4	?	170
vanilla					
dry	0.8 oz	?	1	?	100
prepared	½ c	?	5	?	180

	Portion	Chol (mg)	Total Fat (g)	Satur'd Fat (g)	Total Calor
Instant Sugar-free					
butterscotch, prepared	½ c	?	2	?	100
chocolate					
dry	½ oz	?	0	?	50
prepared	½ c	?	3	?	110
vanilla					
dry	0.4 oz	?	0	?	40
prepared	½ c	?	2	?	100

❏ DESSERTS, FROZEN: ICE CREAM, ICE MILK, ICES & SHERBETS, & FROZEN JUICE, PUDDING, TOFU, & YOGURT

Frozen Pudding on a Stick

banana	1	1	3	3	94
butterscotch	1	1	3	3	94
chocolate	1	1	3	3	99
chocolate fudge	1	1	3	3	99
vanilla	1	1	3	3	93

Frozen Yogurt

IN A CUP

fruit varieties	½ c	?	1	?	108

ON A STICK

plain	1	5	1	?	65
carob/chocolate-coated	1	5	8	?	135
raspberry, chocolate-coated	1	?	7	?	127
strawberry	1	?	1	?	69

Ice Cream

chocolate	1 c	?	16	?	295
French custard	1 c	?	14	?	257
French vanilla, soft serve	1 c	153	23	14	377
strawberry	1 c	?	12	?	250
vanilla					
10% fat	1 c	59	14	9	269
16% fat	1 c	88	24	15	349

	Portion	Chol (mg)	Total Fat (g)	Satur'd Fat (g)	Total Calor
Ice Cream Novelties & Cones					
ice cream cone (cone only)	1	?	tr	?	45
ice cream sandwich	1	?	6	?	167
vanilla ice cream bar w/ chocolate coating	1	?	11	?	162
vanilla ice milk bar w/ chocolate coating	1	?	8	?	144
Ice Milk					
chocolate	⅔ c	?	5	?	137
strawberry	⅔ c	?	3	?	133
vanilla					
regular	1 c	18	6	4	184
soft serve	1 c	13	5	3	223
Ices & Sherbets					
lemon sherbet	¾ c	?	5	?	241
lime/orange ice	1 c	?	tr	?	247
	⅔ c	?	tr	?	165
orange sherbet	1 c	14	4	2	270
sherbet, various flavors	1 c	?	0	0	236
▪ BRAND NAME					
Baskin-Robbins					
CONES					
cake	1	?	tr	?	19
sugar	1	?	1	?	57
ICE CREAM & SHERBET					
chocolate	4 oz	?	13	?	264
Chocolate Mousse Royale	4 oz	?	14	?	293
French vanilla	4 oz	?	19	?	290
orange sherbet	4 oz	?	2	?	158
Pralines 'n Cream	4 oz	?	13	?	283
raspberry sorbet	4 oz	?	0	?	134
Rocky Road	4 oz	?	11	?	291
strawberry	4 oz	?	10	?	226
vanilla	4 oz	?	13	?	235
wild strawberry (low-fat)	4 oz	?	2	?	90
Comet					
cups	1	?	0	?	20
sugar cones	1	?	0	?	40

	Portion	Chol (mg)	Total Fat (g)	Satur'd Fat (g)	Total Calor
Dole					
FRUIT & CREAM BARS					
blueberry	1	?	1	?	90
peach	1	?	1	?	90
strawberry	1	?	1	?	90
FRUIT 'N JUICE BARS					
all flavors except piña colada	1	0	<1	?	70–80
piña colada	1	?	3	?	90
SORBETS					
all flavors	4 oz	0	tr	?	110–120
Drumstick					
Drumstick sundae cone	1	?	10	?	186
Jell-O					
FRUIT BARS					
all flavors	1	0	0	0	45
GELATIN POPS					
all flavors	1	0	0	0	35
PUDDING POPS					
chocolate	1	0	2	?	80
chocolate-covered vanilla	1	0	7	?	130
vanilla w/chocolate chips	1	0	3	?	80
Land O'Lakes					
ice cream, vanilla	4 fl oz	30	7	4	140
ice milk, vanilla	4 fl oz	10	3	2	90
sherbet, fruit flavors	4 fl oz	5	2	1	130
Life Savers					
Flavor Pops, all flavors	1	?	0	?	40
Minute Maid Frozen Fruit Juice Bars					
cherry, fruit punch, grape, orange, strawberry (Variety Pack)	2¼ oz	0	0 or tr	?	60
Snack Pack	1 oz	0	0 or tr	?	25
Oreo Cookies 'n Cream					
ICE CREAM					
chocolate	3 fl oz	?	8	?	140
vanilla	3 fl oz	?	8	?	140
NOVELTIES					
on a stick	1	?	15	?	220
sandwich	1	?	11	?	240
Snackwich	1	?	3	?	60

	Portion	Chol (mg)	Total Fat (g)	Satur'd Fat (g)	Total Calor
Popsicle					
Creamsicle	1	?	3	?	103
Fudgsicle	1	?	tr	?	91
Popsicle	1	0	0	0	65
Tofutti					
LITE LITE					
all flavors	4 oz	0	<1	?	90
PINTS					
Cappuccino Love Drops	4 fl oz	0	12	3	230
Chocolate Love Drops	4 fl oz	0	13	5	230
Chocolate Supreme	4 fl oz	0	13	3	210
vanilla	4 fl oz	0	11	2	200
vanilla almond bark	4 fl oz	0	14	3	230
Vanilla Love Drops	4 fl oz	0	12	3	220
wildberry	4 fl oz	0	12	2	210
SINGLE SERVINGS					
Chocolate Cuties	1	0	5	2	140
Vanilla Cuties	1	0	5	1	130
SOFT SERVE					
regular	4 fl oz	0	8	2	158
Hi-Lite					
chocolate	4 fl oz	0	1	tr	100
vanilla	4 fl oz	0	1	tr	90

❑ DESSERT SAUCES, SYRUPS, & TOPPINGS

See also NUTS & NUT-BASED BUTTERS, FLOURS, MEALS, MILKS, PASTES, & POWDERS

Sauces, Syrups, & Flavored Toppings

	Portion	Chol (mg)	Total Fat (g)	Satur'd Fat (g)	Total Calor
butterscotch sauce, home-made	2 T	?	7	?	203
butterscotch topping	3 T	?	tr	?	156
caramel topping	3 T	?	tr	?	155
cherry topping	3 T	?	tr	?	147
chocolate-flavored syrup or topping					
fudge type	2 T	0	5	3	125
thin type	2 T	0	tr	tr	85
custard sauce, homemade	4 T	?	4	?	85
hard sauce, homemade	4 T	?	11	?	193
honey *See* SUGARS & SWEETENERS					

	Portion	Chol (mg)	Total Fat (g)	Satur'd Fat (g)	Total Calor
lemon sauce, homemade	4 T	?	3	?	133
pineapple topping	3 T	?	tr	?	146
walnuts in syrup topping	3 T	?	1	?	169

Whipped Cream & Whipped Cream–Type Toppings

	Portion	Chol (mg)	Total Fat (g)	Satur'd Fat (g)	Total Calor
nondairy					
powdered, prepared w/	1 T	tr	1	tr	8
whole milk	1 c	8	10	9	151
pressurized, containing	1 T	0	1	1	11
lauric acid oil & sodium caseinate	1 c	0	16	13	184
semisolid, frozen, containing lauric acid oil & sodium caseinate	1 T	0	1	1	13
	1 c	0	19	16	239
whipped cream topping, pressurized	1 T	2	1	4	8
	1 c	46	13	8	154

▪ BRAND NAME

	Portion	Chol (mg)	Total Fat (g)	Satur'd Fat (g)	Total Calor
Cool Whip					
Extra Creamy Dairy Recipe whipped topping	1 T	0	1	?	16
nondairy whipped topping	1 T	0	1	?	12
Dream Whip					
whipped topping mix, prepared w/whole milk	1 T	0	0	0	10
D-Zerta					
reduced-calorie whipped topping	1 T	0	1	?	8
Featherweight					
whipped topping	1 T	?	0	?	2
Hershey					
chocolate fudge topping	2 T	?	4	?	100
Smucker's					
butterscotch	2 T	?	1	?	140
caramel	2 T	?	1	?	140
chocolate fudge	2 T	?	1	?	130
fruit syrups	2 T	?	0	0	100
hot caramel	2 T	?	4	?	150
hot fudge	2 T	?	4	?	110
peanut butter caramel	2 T	?	2	?	150
pineapple	2 T	?	0	0	130
strawberry	2 T	?	0	0	120
walnuts in syrup	2 T	?	1	?	130

	Portion	Chol (mg)	Total Fat (g)	Satur'd Fat (g)	Total Calor

❑ DINNERS, FROZEN

▪ BRAND NAME

Health Valley Lean Living

	Portion	Chol (mg)	Total Fat (g)	Satur'd Fat (g)	Total Calor
cheese enchiladas	9 oz	?	5	?	280
chicken à la king	9 oz	?	17	?	380
chicken crêpes	9 oz	?	22	?	380
spinach lasagna	9 oz	?	3	?	170

Hungry-Man Dinners *See* Swanson, *below*
Lean Cuisine *See* Stouffer, *below*
Le Menu

	Portion	Chol (mg)	Total Fat (g)	Satur'd Fat (g)	Total Calor
beef sirloin tips	11½ oz	?	19	?	410
beef Stroganoff	10 oz	?	26	?	450
breast of chicken parmigiana	11½ oz	?	19	?	390
chicken à la king	10¼ oz	?	13	?	330
chicken cordon bleu	11 oz	?	20	?	470
chicken Florentine	12½ oz	?	24	?	480
chopped sirloin beef	12¼ oz	?	19	?	410
ham steak	10 oz	?	11	?	310
pepper steak	11½ oz	?	14	?	380
sliced breast of turkey w/ mushrooms	11¼ oz	?	23	?	460
stuffed flounder	10¼ oz	?	18	?	350
sweet & sour chicken	11¼ oz	?	23	?	460
vegetable lasagna	11 oz	?	19	?	360
Yankee pot roast	11 oz	?	15	?	360

Le Menu Light Style

	Portion	Chol (mg)	Total Fat (g)	Satur'd Fat (g)	Total Calor
beef à l'orange	10 oz	?	8	?	290
chicken cacciatore	10 oz	?	8	?	260
flounder vin blanc	10 oz	?	5	?	220
glazed chicken breast	10 oz	?	5	?	240
3-cheese stuffed shells	10 oz	?	8	?	280
turkey divan	10 oz	?	9	?	280

L'Orient

	Portion	Chol (mg)	Total Fat (g)	Satur'd Fat (g)	Total Calor
beef broccoli	11 oz	?	30	?	530
Cantonese chicken chow mein	11½ oz	?	5	?	280
Firecracker chicken	10½ oz	?	10	?	380
lemon chicken	11 oz	?	15	?	400
orange beef	10¾ oz	?	12	?	380
rock sugar–glazed pork	10¾ oz	?	15	?	360

	Portion	Chol (mg)	Total Fat (g)	Satur'd Fat (g)	Total Calor
Stouffer					
DINNER SUPREME					
baked chicken breast w/ gravy	11 oz	?	9	?	330
beef teriyaki	11⅜ oz	?	13	?	370
beef tips Bourguignonne	12⅜ oz	?	15	?	360
chicken Florentine	11 oz	?	18	?	430
chicken w/Supreme Sauce	11⅜ oz	?	12	?	360
flounder w/dill cream sauce	11⅝ oz	?	19	?	370
flounder w/roasted red pepper sauce	12 oz	?	19	?	360
Salisbury steak w/gravy & mushrooms	13½ oz	?	18	?	380
LEAN CUISINE					
beef & pork cannelloni w/ Mornay sauce	9⅝ oz	50	10	?	270
breast of chicken Marsala w/vegetables	8⅛ oz	60	5	?	190
cheese cannelloni w/to-mato sauce	9⅛ oz	35	10	?	270
chicken à l'orange w/al-mond rice	8 oz	55	5	?	270
chicken & vegetables w/ vermicelli	12¾ oz	50	7	?	270
chicken cacciatore w/ver-micelli	10⅞ oz	55	10	?	280
chicken chow mein w/rice	11¼ oz	35	5	?	250
filet of fish divan	12⅜ oz	95	9	?	270
filet of fish Florentine	9 oz	90	9	?	240
filet of fish jardiniere w/ souffléed potatoes	11¼ oz	110	10	?	280
glazed chicken w/vegetable rice	8½ oz	65	8	?	270
herbed lamb w/rice	10⅜ oz	70	8	?	280
linguini w/clam sauce	9⅝ oz	35	7	?	260
meatball stew	10 oz	80	10	?	250
Oriental beef w/vegetables & rice	8⅝ oz	45	8	?	270
Oriental scallops & vegeta-bles w/rice	11 oz	20	3	?	220
Salisbury steak w/Italian-style sauce & vegeta-bles	9½ oz	110	13	?	270
shrimp & chicken Can-tonese w/noodles	10⅛ oz	130	9	?	270
spaghetti w/beef & mush-room sauce	11½ oz	30	7	?	280

	Portion	Chol (mg)	Total Fat (g)	Satur'd Fat (g)	Total Calor
stuffed cabbage w/meat in tomato sauce	10¾ oz	45	9	?	220
tuna lasagna w/spinach noodles & vegetables	9¾ oz	25	10	?	280
turkey Dijon	9½ oz	70	10	?	280
veal lasagna	10¼ oz	90	8	?	280
veal primavera	9⅛ oz	90	9	?	250
zucchini lasagna	11 oz	25	7	?	260

Swanson
3-COMPARTMENT DINNERS

beans & franks	10½ oz	?	17	?	420
macaroni & beef	12 oz	?	15	?	370
macaroni & cheese	12¼ oz	?	15	?	380
noodles & chicken	10½ oz	?	9	?	270
spaghetti & meatballs	12½ oz	?	15	?	370

4-COMPARTMENT DINNERS

beans & franks	10½ oz	?	20	?	500
beef enchiladas	13¾ oz	?	24	?	480
chicken in barbecue sauce	11¾ oz	?	13	?	450
chicken nugget platter	8¾ oz	?	25	?	470
chopped sirloin beef	11 oz	?	20	?	380
fish & chips	10 oz	?	20	?	500
fish nugget	9½ oz	?	23	?	450
fried chicken					
barbecue-flavored	edible portion = 10 oz	?	27	?	580
dark meat	edible portion = 10 oz	?	28	?	580
white meat	edible portion = 10½ oz	?	27	?	580
loin of pork	10¾ oz	?	12	?	310
meat loaf	10¾ oz	?	21	?	430
Mexican-style combination	14¼ oz	?	25	?	500
Polynesian style	12 oz	?	8	?	360
Salisbury steak	10¾ oz	?	18	?	410
sweet & sour chicken	12 oz	?	13	?	390
Swiss steak	10 oz	?	11	?	350
turkey	11½ oz	?	11	?	360
veal parmigiana	12¼ oz	?	23	?	460
Western style	11½ oz	?	21	?	440

HUNGRY-MAN DINNERS

boneless chicken	17¾ oz	?	27	?	710
chicken nuggets	16 oz	?	26	?	600
chicken parmigiana	20 oz	?	51	?	810
chopped beef steak	16¾ oz	?	33	?	590

	Portion	Chol (mg)	Total Fat (g)	Satur'd Fat (g)	Total Calor
fish & chips	14¾ oz	?	39	?	780
fried chicken					
breast portions	14½ oz	?	50	?	930
dark portions	edible portion = 14½ oz	?	48	?	910
lasagna	18¾ oz	?	26	?	740
Mexican style	20¼ oz	?	39	?	750
Salisbury steak	18¼ oz	?	42	?	660
sliced beef	15½ oz	?	13	?	470
turkey	17 oz	?	18	?	550
veal parmigiana	18¼ oz	?	30	?	630
Western style	17½ oz	?	34	?	740

▢ EGGS & EGG SUBSTITUTES

Chicken Eggs

COOKED

egg dishes, prepared *See* BREAKFAST FOODS, PREPARED; FAST FOODS

	Portion	Chol (mg)	Total Fat (g)	Satur'd Fat (g)	Total Calor
fried in butter	1 large	246	6	2	83
hard boiled	1 large	274	6	2	79
omelet, cooked w/butter & milk	1 egg (large)	248	7	3	95
poached	1 large	273	6	2	79
scrambled, w/butter & milk	1 large	248	7	3	95

DRIED

	Portion	Chol (mg)	Total Fat (g)	Satur'd Fat (g)	Total Calor
whole	1 c sifted	1,631	36	11	505
whole, stabilized (glucose-reduced)	1 c sifted	1,714	37	11	523
white only					
flakes, stabilized (glucose-reduced)	½ lb	0	tr	0	796
powder, stabilized (glucose-reduced)	1 c sifted	0	tr	0	402
yolk only	1 c sifted	1,962	41	12	460

UNCOOKED

	Portion	Chol (mg)	Total Fat (g)	Satur'd Fat (g)	Total Calor
whole, fresh or frozen	1	274	6	2	79
white only, fresh or frozen	1	0	tr	0	16
yolk only, fresh	1	272	6	2	63

Eggs, Other

	Portion	Chol (mg)	Total Fat (g)	Satur'd Fat (g)	Total Calor
duck	1	619	10	3	130
goose	1	?	19	5	267

	Portion	Chol (mg)	Total Fat (g)	Satur'd Fat (g)	Total Calor
quail	1	76	1	tr	14
turkey	1	737	9	3	135

Egg Substitute

frozen, containing egg white, corn oil, & non-fat dry milk	¼ c	1	7	1	96
liquid, containing egg white, soybean oil, & soy protein	1 c	3	8	2	211
powder, containing egg white solids, whole egg solids, sweet whey solids, nonfat dry milk, & soy protein	0.7 oz	113	3	1	88

▪ BRAND NAME

Featherweight

egg substitute	2 eggs	?	8	?	120
Fleischmann's					
Egg Beaters	¼ c	0	0	?	25
Egg Beaters w/Cheez	½ c	5	6	?	130
Oregon Freeze Dry					
cheese omelet	2 eggs	?	12	?	240
eggs, w/butter	2 eggs	?	9	?	183
precooked eggs, w/real bacon	2 eggs	?	12	?	180

❑ ENTREES & MAIN COURSES, CANNED & BOXED

chili & bean products, canned & boxed *See* LEGUMES & LEGUME PRODUCTS; SOYBEANS & SOYBEAN PRODUCTS

▪ BRAND NAME

Armour Star

beef stew	7½ oz	?	11	?	210
corned & roast beef hash & sloppy joes *See* PROCESSED MEAT & POULTRY PRODUCTS					

	Portion	Chol (mg)	Total Fat (g)	Satur'd Fat (g)	Total Calor
Chun King					
DIVIDER PAK ENTREES, CANNED					
4 Servings/42 Oz Pkg					
beef chow mein	7 oz	15	2	1	100
beef pepper Oriental	7 oz	15	4	1	110
chicken chow mein	7 oz	15	4	2	110
pork chow mein	7 oz	25	4	0	120
shrimp chow mein	7 oz	30	2	0	100
2 Servings/24 Oz Pkg					
beef chow mein	8 oz	20	2	1	110
chicken chow mein	8 oz	10	4	1	120
STIR-FRY ENTREES, CANNED					
chow mein w/beef	6 oz	50	19	4	290
chow mein w/chicken	6 oz	45	11	6	220
egg foo young	5 oz	140	8	2	140
pepper steak	6 oz	50	17	4	250
sukiyaki	6 oz	50	17	3	260
Featherweight					
beef ravioli	8 oz	?	4	?	220
beef stew	7½ oz	?	8	?	220
boned chicken	13 oz	?	11	?	186
chicken stew	7½ oz	?	6	?	170
chicken w/dumplings	7½ oz	?	5	?	160
spaghetti w/meatballs	7½ oz	?	5	?	200
Franco-American					
beef ravioli in meat sauce	7½ oz	?	5	?	230
macaroni & cheese	7⅜ oz	?	5	?	170
PizzO's	7½ oz	?	2	?	170
spaghetti in tomato sauce w/cheese	7⅜ oz	?	2	?	190
SpaghettiO's in tomato & cheese sauce	7⅜ oz	?	2	?	170
spaghetti w/meatballs in tomato sauce	7⅜ oz	?	8	?	220
Noodle-Roni Pasta					
chicken & mushroom flavor, prepared	½ c	?	3	?	150
fettucini, prepared	½ c	?	17	?	300
garlic & butter, prepared	½ c	?	16	?	290
herbs & butter, prepared	½ c	?	7	?	160
parmesano, prepared	½ c	?	13	?	230
pesto Italiano, prepared	½ c	?	11	?	210
Rominoff, prepared	½ c	?	11	?	240
Stroganoff, prepared	¾ c	?	19	?	360
Swanson					
chicken à la king	5¼ oz	?	12	?	180
chicken & dumplings	7½ oz	?	12	?	220
chicken stew	7⅝ oz	?	7	?	170

	Portion	Chol (mg)	Total Fat (g)	Satur'd Fat (g)	Total Calor
Van Camp's					
Noodle Weenee	1 c	?	9	?	245
tamales w/sauce	1 c	?	16	?	293

❑ ENTREES & MAIN COURSES, FROZEN

Celentano

	Portion	Chol (mg)	Total Fat (g)	Satur'd Fat (g)	Total Calor
baked pasta & cheese	12 oz	75	21	?	530
broccoli stuffed shells	11½ oz	?	17	?	400
cannelloni Florentine	12 oz	?	17	?	380
cavatelli	3.2 oz	?	1	?	270
chicken cutlets parmigiana	9 oz	?	5	?	310
chicken primavera	11½ oz	?	9	?	270
eggplant parmigiana	8 oz	?	22	?	330
	7 oz	?	12	?	270
Eggplant Rollettes	11 oz	?	30	?	420
lasagne	8 oz	?	16	?	320
	6¼ oz	?	7	?	250
lasagne primavera	11 oz	?	9	?	300
manicotti					
w/sauce	8 oz	?	15	?	300
w/out sauce	7 oz	?	18	?	380
ravioli					
miniround cheese, w/out sauce	4 oz	?	6	?	250
round cheese, w/out sauce	6½ oz	?	12	?	410
stuffed shells					
w/sauce	8 oz	?	14	?	320
w/out sauce	6¼ oz	?	15	?	350

Lean Cuisine See Stouffer, *under* DINNERS, FROZEN

Le Menu Entrees

	Portion	Chol (mg)	Total Fat (g)	Satur'd Fat (g)	Total Calor
beef burgundy	7½ oz	?	23	?	330
chicken Kiev	8 oz	?	39	?	530
manicotti	8½ oz	?	12	?	300
Oriental chicken	8½ oz	?	6	?	260

Mrs. Paul's

eggplant parmigiana See VEGETABLES, PLAIN & PREPARED

AU NATUREL SEAFOOD

	Portion	Chol (mg)	Total Fat (g)	Satur'd Fat (g)	Total Calor
cod fillets	4 oz	?	2	?	90
flounder fillets	4 oz	?	2	?	90
haddock fillets	4 oz	?	1	?	80
perch fillets	4 oz	?	2	?	80
sole fillets	4 oz	?	2	?	90

	Portion	Chol (mg)	Total Fat (g)	Satur'd Fat (g)	Total Calor
BUTTERED SEAFOOD					
fish fillets	2	?	9	?	170
LIGHT SEAFOOD ENTREES					
fish & pasta Florentine	9½ oz	?	9	?	240
fish au gratin	10 oz	?	8	?	290
fish Dijon	9½ oz	?	15	?	280
fish Florentine	9 oz	?	4	?	210
fish Mornay	10 oz	?	14	?	280
shrimp & clams w/linguini	10 oz	?	6	?	280
shrimp Cajun style	10½ oz	?	4	?	200
shrimp Oriental	11 oz	?	5	?	280
shrimp primavera	11 oz	?	4	?	240
tuna pasta casserole	11 oz	?	7	?	290
PREPARED BATTERED SEAFOOD					
batter-dipped fish fillets	2	?	25	?	390
Crunchy Light Batter					
fish fillets	2	?	17	?	310
fish sticks	4	?	13	?	240
flounder fillets	2	?	16	?	310
haddock fillets	2	?	17	?	330
fried clams in a light batter	2½ oz	?	13	?	240
PREPARED BREADED SEAFOOD					
catfish fillets	1	?	10	?	220
combination seafood platter	9 oz	?	31	?	590
Crispy Crunchy					
fish fillets	2	?	16	?	280
fish sticks	4	?	10	?	200
flounder fillets	2	?	15	?	270
haddock fillets	2	?	12	?	250
perch fillets	2	?	19	?	320
deviled crabs	1 piece	?	8	?	190
fish cakes	2	?	11	?	250
french-fried scallops	3½ oz	?	9	?	230
fried shrimp	3 oz	?	11	?	200
Supreme Light Breaded					
fish fillets	1	?	13	?	290
flounder or sole fillets	1	?	13	?	280
Sara Lee Le Sandwich Croissants					
cheddar cheese	1	?	23	?	380
chicken & broccoli	1	?	17	?	340
ham & Swiss cheese	1	?	18	?	340
turkey, bacon, & cheese	1	?	20	?	370

	Portion	Chol (mg)	Total Fat (g)	Satur'd Fat (g)	Total Calor
Stouffer					
ENTREES					
beef & spinach stuffed pasta shells w/tomato sauce	9 oz	?	12	?	300
beef chop suey w/rice	12 oz	?	12	?	340
beef pie	10 oz	?	37	?	560
beef stew	10 oz	?	16	?	310
beef Stroganoff w/parsley noodles	9¾ oz	?	21	?	410
beef teriyaki in sauce w/ rice & vegetables	9¾ oz	?	9	?	330
cashew chicken in sauce w/rice	9½ oz	?	17	?	410
cheese soufflé	7⅝ oz	?	36	?	480
cheese stuffed pasta shells w/meat sauce	9 oz	?	16	?	340
chicken à la king w/rice	9½ oz	?	11	?	320
chicken chow mein w/out noodles	8 oz	?	5	?	140
chicken crêpes w/mushroom sauce	8¼ oz	?	21	?	370
chicken divan	8½ oz	?	22	?	350
chicken paprikash w/egg noodles	10½ oz	?	15	?	390
chicken pie	10 oz	?	34	?	530
chicken stuffed pasta shells w/cheese sauce	9 oz	?	24	?	420
chili con carne w/beans	8¾ oz	?	11	?	280
creamed chicken	6½ oz	?	24	?	320
creamed chipped beef	5½ oz	?	17	?	240
escalloped chicken & noodles	5¾ oz	?	16	?	260
fettucini Alfredo	5 oz	?	20	?	280
fettucini primavera	½ of 10⅝ oz pkg	?	21	?	270
green pepper steak w/rice	10½ oz	?	11	?	340
Ham & Asparagus Bake	9½ oz	?	35	?	510
ham & asparagus crêpes	6¼ oz	?	18	?	310
ham & Swiss cheese crêpes w/cream sauce	7½ oz	?	26	?	410
lasagna	10½ oz	?	13	?	370
linguini w/pesto sauce	½ of 8¼ oz pkg	?	10	?	210
lobster Newburg	6½ oz	?	30	?	360
macaroni & beef w/tomatoes	11½ oz	?	16	?	360
macaroni & cheese	6 oz	?	12	?	250
noodles Romanoff	4 oz	?	9	?	170
roast beef hash	5¾ oz	?	15	?	250

	Portion	Chol (mg)	Total Fat (g)	Satur'd Fat (g)	Total Calor
Salisbury steaks w/onion gravy	6 oz	?	14	?	230
Scallops & Shrimp Mariner w/Rice	10¼ oz	?	18	?	390
short ribs of beef w/vegetable gravy	5¾ oz	?	20	?	280
spaghetti w/meatballs	12⅝ oz	?	13	?	370
spaghetti w/meat sauce	14 oz	?	15	?	440
spinach crêpes w/cheddar cheese sauce	9½ oz	?	27	?	420
steak & mushroom pie	10 oz	?	24	?	430
stuffed green peppers w/ beef in tomato sauce	7¾ oz	?	11	?	220
Swedish meatballs in gravy w/parsley noodles	11 oz	?	25	?	470
tuna noodle casserole	5¾ oz	?	8	?	190
turkey casserole w/gravy & dressing	9¾ oz	?	19	?	380
turkey pie	10 oz	?	35	?	540
turkey tetrazzini	6 oz	?	14	?	230
vegetable lasagna	10½ oz	?	25	?	450
Welsh rarebit	5 oz	?	30	?	360

LEAN CUISINE See Stouffer, *under* DINNERS, FROZEN

Swanson
CHICKEN DUET ENTREES

creamy broccoli	6 oz	?	17	?	310
creamy green bean	6 oz	?	18	?	330
saucy tomato	6 oz	?	18	?	340
savory wild rice	6 oz	?	14	?	290

CHICKEN DUET GOURMET NUGGETS

ham & cheese	3 oz	?	13	?	220
Mexican style	3 oz	?	13	?	220
pizza style	3 oz	?	12	?	210
spinach & herb	3 oz	?	13	?	230

CHUNKY PIES

beef	10 oz	?	29	?	550
chicken	10 oz	?	33	?	580
turkey	10 oz	?	31	?	540

DIPSTERS

barbecue	3 oz	?	13	?	220
Coconola	3 oz	?	15	?	240
herb	3 oz	?	14	?	220
Italian style	3 oz	?	16	?	230

	Portion	Chol (mg)	Total Fat (g)	Satur'd Fat (g)	Total Calor
ENTREES					
Chicken Nibbles	edible portion = 5 oz	?	18	?	260
Fish 'n' Fries	7¼ oz	?	21	?	420
fried chicken	edible portion = 6½ oz	?	19	?	300
Salisbury steak	10 oz	?	32	?	410
Swedish meatballs	9¼ oz	?	30	?	420
turkey	8¾ oz	?	11	?	270
veal parmigiana	10 oz	?	15	?	280
HUNGRY-MAN POT PIES					
beef	16 oz	?	33	?	680
chicken	16 oz	?	41	?	730
turkey	16 oz	?	38	?	690
MAIN COURSE ENTREES					
lasagna w/meat	13¼ oz	?	19	?	470
macaroni & cheese	12 oz	?	16	?	390
PLUMP & JUICY					
chicken cutlets	3 oz	?	12	?	200
Chicken Dipsters	3 oz	?	14	?	220
Chicken Drumlets	3 oz	?	14	?	220
Chicken Nibbles	3¼ oz	?	20	?	300
Extra Crispy fried chicken	3 oz	?	16	?	250
fried chicken					
assorted pieces	3¼ oz	?	17	?	270
breast portions	4½ oz	?	21	?	360
Take-Out fried chicken, assorted pieces	3¼ oz	?	17	?	270
thighs & drumsticks	3¼ oz	?	19	?	280
POT PIES					
beef	8 oz	?	21	?	410
chicken	8 oz	?	26	?	420
macaroni & cheese	7 oz	?	9	?	220
turkey	8 oz	?	24	?	410
Tyson					
chicken cordon bleu	about 3½ oz	38	13	1	225
chicken Kiev	about 3½ oz	73	22	2	290
stuffed chicken breast	about 3½ oz	34	7	1	160

	Portion	Chol (mg)	Total Fat (g)	Satur'd Fat (g)	Total Calor

□ FAST FOODS

shakes					
chocolate	10 fl oz	37	11	7	360
strawberry	10 fl oz	31	8	?	319
vanilla	10 fl oz	32	8	5	314
tacos	1	21	11	4	195

▪ BRAND NAME

Arby's
CHICKEN, ROASTED

	Portion	Chol (mg)	Total Fat (g)	Satur'd Fat (g)	Total Calor
breast	1	200	7	?	254
leg	1	214	16	?	319

DESSERTS

apple turnover	1	0	18	7	303
cherry turnover	1	0	18	5	280

SALADS

chicken salad & croissant	1	12	36	?	472
chicken salad w/tomato & lettuce	1	12	36	?	515
tossed salad					
plain	1	0	tr	?	44
w/low-cal Italian dressing	1	0	1	?	57

SANDWICHES

Bac'n Cheddar Deluxe	1	83	37	10	526
Beef'n Cheddar	1	63	27	8	455
chicken breast	1	83	29	6	509
chicken club	1	108	32	?	621
chicken salad	1	30	20	?	386
fish fillet	1	70	32	10	580
hot ham & cheese	1	45	14	5	292
Philly Beef 'n Swiss	1	107	28	10	460
roast beef					
junior	1	20	9	4	218
regular	1	39	15	7	353
king	1	49	19	9	467
giant	1	65	23	12	531
super	1	40	22	9	501
Turkey Deluxe	1	39	17	4	375

	Portion	Chol (mg)	Total Fat (g)	Satur'd Fat (g)	Total Calor
SHAKES					
chocolate	1	36	12	3	451
Jamocha	1	35	11	3	368
vanilla	1	32	12	4	330
SIDE DISHES					
french fries	1 serving	8	10	5	215
potato cakes	1 serving	13	13	7	201
rice pilaf	1 serving	0	2	?	123
Scandinavian vegetables in sauce	1 serving	0	2	?	56
Burger King					
BREAKFAST ITEMS					
Breakfast Croissan'wich	1	243	19	6	304
w/bacon	1	249	24	8	355
w/ham	1	262	20	6	335
w/sausage	1	293	41	14	538
French toast sticks	1 serving	74	29	5	499
Great Danish	1	6	36	23	500
scrambled egg platter	1	370	30	?	468
w/bacon	1	378	36	?	536
w/sausage	1	420	52	?	702
BURGERS & SANDWICHES					
bacon double cheeseburger	1	104	31	15	510
cheeseburger	1	48	15	7	317
Chicken Specialty	1	82	40	8	688
Ham & Cheese Specialty	1	70	23	9	471
hamburger	1	37	12	5	275
Whaler fish	1	77	27	6	488
Whopper	1	90	36	12	628
w/cheese	1	113	43	17	711
Whopper Jr.	1	41	17	6	322
w/cheese	1	52	20	8	364
CHICKEN					
Chicken Tenders	6 pieces	47	10	2	204
DESSERTS					
apple pie	1 slice	4	12	4	305
SALADS					
plain salad	1 serving	0	0	0	28
w/bleu cheese dressing	1 serving	22	16	3	184
w/house dressing	1 serving	11	13	2	158
w/reduced-calorie Italian dressing	1 serving	0	0	0	42
w/Thousand Island dressing	1 serving	17	12	2	145

	Portion	Chol (mg)	Total Fat (g)	Satur'd Fat (g)	Total Calor
SHAKES					
chocolate	1 regular	?	12	?	320
syrup added	1 regular	?	11	?	374
vanilla	1 regular	?	10	?	321
syrup added	1 regular	?	10	?	334
SIDE DISHES					
french fries	1 regular serving	14	13	7	227
onion rings	1 regular serving	0	16	3	274
Church's Fried Chicken					
CHICKEN					
breast	1	?	17	?	278
leg	1	?	9	?	147
thigh	1	?	22	?	306
wing-breast	1	?	20	?	303
SIDE DISHES					
corn, w/butter oil	1 ear	?	9	?	237
french fries, w/salt	1 regular serving	?	6	?	138
Hardee's					
BREAKFAST ITEMS					
American cheese slice	1	12	3	?	47
bacon & egg biscuit	1	338	26	?	410
Big Country Breakfast bacon	1 serving	350	50	?	761
Big Country Breakfast ham	1 serving	369	38	?	665
Big Country Breakfast sausage	1 serving	442	70	?	849
biscuit gravy	1 serving	21	10	?	144
Canadian Sunrise biscuit	1	249	30	?	482
cinnamon & raisin biscuit	1	0	16	?	276
cheese biscuit	1	12	16	?	304
country ham biscuit	1	12	18	?	323
egg	1	143	6	?	79
egg biscuit	1	143	19	?	336
ham biscuit	1	17	14	?	300
Hash Rounds potatoes	1 serving	9	16	?	249
jam	1 serving	0	0	0	51
Rise 'n' Shine biscuit	1	0	12	?	257
sausage & egg biscuit	1	179	35	?	503
sausage biscuit	1	25	28	?	426
steak biscuit	1	16	28	?	491

	Portion	Chol (mg)	Total Fat (g)	Satur'd Fat (g)	Total Calor
BURGERS & SANDWICHES					
bacon cheeseburger	1	60	33	?	556
big deluxe burger	1	54	29	?	503
cheeseburger					
regular	1	31	15	?	327
¼ lb	1	77	28	?	511
chicken fillet	1	59	17	?	446
Fisherman's Fillet	1	80	20	?	469
hamburger	1	20	9	?	244
hot dog	1	0	14	?	285
hot ham & cheese	1	57	10	?	316
mushroom & Swiss burger	1	86	23	?	509
roast beef					
regular	1	68	12	?	312
big	1	86	22	?	440
turkey club	1	45	22	?	426
DESSERTS					
apple turnover	1	0	13	?	87
Big Cookie Treat	1	9	15	?	54
Cool Twist cone	1	18	5	?	164
SALADS					
chef salad	1	172	13	?	309
garden salad, w/Thousand Island dressing	1	290	34	?	501
side salad	1	0	tr	?	90
SHAKES					
chocolate	1	42	10	?	390
SIDE DISHES					
french fries	1 regular serving	0	12	?	252
	1 large serving	0	23	?	438
Jack-in-the-Box					
BEVERAGES					
hot chocolate	1	tr	4	tr	133
BREAKFAST ITEMS					
Breakfast Jack	1	203	13	5	307
grape jelly	1 serving	0	0	0	38
pancake platter	1	99	22	9	612
pancake syrup	1 serving	0	0	0	121
scrambled egg platter	1	354	40	17	662

	Portion	Chol (mg)	Total Fat (g)	Satur'd Fat (g)	Total Calor
BURGERS & SANDWICHES					
bacon cheeseburger	1	85	39	15	705
cheeseburger	1	41	17	8	325
Chicken Supreme	1	62	36	14	575
club pita, w/out sauce	1	43	8	4	277
ham & Swiss burger	1	106	49	21	754
hamburger	1	26	13	5	288
Hot Club Supreme	1	82	28	9	524
Jumbo Jack	1	73	34	11	584
w/cheese	1	102	40	14	677
Moby Jack	1	47	25	8	444
Monterey burger	1	152	57	28	808
mushroom burger	1	64	24	10	513
Swiss & bacon burger	1	92	·47	20	678
Ultimate Cheeseburger	1	127	69	26	942
CRESCENT ROLLS					
Canadian crescent	1	226	31	10	452
sausage crescent	1	187	43	16	584
Supreme crescent	1	178	40	13	547
DESSERTS					
cheesecake	1 piece	63	18	9	309
hot apple turnover	1	15	24	11	410
ENTREES					
chicken strip dinner	1	86	29	13	674
shrimp dinner	1	128	33	15	677
sirloin steak dinner	1	56	27	9	702
MEXICAN DISHES					
Fajita Pita	1	30	7	3	278
guacamole	1 serving	0	5	tr	55
nachos					
cheese	1 serving	37	35	13	571
Supreme	1 serving	59	45	17	787
salsa	1 serving	0	<1	<1	8
taco	1	21	11	5	191
Super taco	1	37	17	8	288
PIZZA					
Pizza Pocket	1	32	28	13	497
SALAD DRESSINGS					
bleu cheese	1 serving	9	11	2	131
buttermilk house	1 serving	10	18	3	181
reduced-calorie French	1 serving	0	4	1	80
Thousand Island	1 serving	11	15	3	156

	Portion	Chol (mg)	Total Fat (g)	Satur'd Fat (g)	Total Calor
SALADS					
chef salad	1	107	18	9	295
pasta & seafood salad	1	48	22	4	394
side salad	1	<1	3	2	51
taco salad	1	102	24	10	377
SAUCES					
A-1 Steak	1 serving	0	<1	<1	18
BBQ	1 serving	0	<1	<1	39
Mayo-Mustard	1 serving	10	13	<1	124
Mayo-Onion	1 serving	20	15	tr	143
Seafood Cocktail	1 serving	0	<1	<1	57
SHAKES					
chocolate	1	25	7	4	330
strawberry	1	25	7	4	320
vanilla	1	25	6	4	320
SIDE DISHES					
french fries	1 regular serving	8	12	5	221
	1 large serving	13	19	8	353
onion rings	1 serving	27	23	11	382

Kentucky Fried Chicken
FRIED CHICKEN

Original Recipe

	Portion	Chol (mg)	Total Fat (g)	Satur'd Fat (g)	Total Calor
breast					
center	1	93	14	4	257
side	1	96	17	5	276
drumstick	1	81	9	2	147
thigh	1	122	19	5	278
wing	1	67	12	3	181
Extra Crispy					
breast					
center	1	93	21	5	353
side	1	66	24	6	354
drumstick	1	65	11	3	173
thigh	1	121	26	7	371
wing	1	63	16	4	218
NUGGETS & SAUCES					
nuggets	1	12	3	1	46
barbecue sauce	1 oz	<1	1	<1	35
honey sauce	½ oz	<1	<1	<1	49
mustard sauce	1 oz	<1	1	<1	36
sweet & sour sauce	1 oz	<1	1	<1	58

	Portion	Chol (mg)	Total Fat (g)	Satur'd Fat (g)	Total Calor
SIDE DISHES					
baked beans	1 serving	<1	1	tr	105
buttermilk biscuits	1	<1	14	3	269
chicken gravy	1 serving	2	4	1	59
cole slaw	1 serving	4	6	1	103
corn on the cob	1 ear	<1	3	1	176
Kentucky fries	1 serving	2	13	3	268
mashed potatoes	1 serving	<1	1	tr	59
w/gravy	1 serving	<1	1	tr	62
potato salad	1 serving	11	9	1	141
McDonald's					
BREAKFAST ITEMS					
biscuit					
w/bacon, cheese, & egg	1	263	32	9	483
w/biscuit spread	1	9	18	8	330
w/sausage	1	48	31	12	467
w/sausage & egg	1	285	40	15	585
danish					
apple	1	26	18	3	389
cinnamon raisin	1	35	21	4	445
iced cheese	1	48	22	6	395
raspberry	1	27	16	3	414
Egg McMuffin	1	259	16	6	340
English muffin w/butter	1	15	5	2	186
hash brown potatoes	1 serving	7	9	4	144
hotcakes w/butter syrup	1 serving	47	10	4	500
pork sausage	1 serving	39	19	7	210
Sausage McMuffin	1	59	26	10	427
w/egg	1	287	33	13	517
scrambled eggs	1 serving	514	13	5	180
BURGERS & SANDWICHES					
Big Mac	1	83	35	12	570
cheeseburger	1	41	16	7	318
Filet-o-Fish	1	47	26	6	435
hamburger	1	29	11	4	263
McD.L.T.	1	101	44	15	680
Quarter Pounder	1	81	24	9	427
w/cheese	1	107	32	13	525
CHICKEN NUGGETS & SAUCES					
Chicken McNuggets	2	63	20	5	323
barbecue sauce	1 serving	tr	tr	tr	60
honey	1 serving	tr	tr	tr	50
hot mustard sauce	1 serving	3	2	tr	63
sweet & sour sauce	1 serving	tr	tr	tr	64

	Portion	Chol (mg)	Total Fat (g)	Satur'd Fat (g)	Total Calor
DESSERTS					
apple pie	1 piece	7	14	5	253
cookies					
Chocolaty Chip	1 serving	18	16	8	342
McDonaldland	1 serving	10	11	4	308
soft-serve ice cream & cone	1 serving	24	5	2	189
sundaes					
hot caramel	1	31	10	3	361
hot fudge	1	27	11	5	357
strawberry	1	25	9	3	320
SALAD BAR ITEMS					
bacon bits	1 serving	3	1	tr	15
chef salad	1	125	13	6	226
chicken salad Oriental	1	92	4	1	146
chow mein noodles	1 serving	2	2	tr	45
croutons	1 serving	1	2	tr	52
garden salad	1	110	6	3	91
shrimp salad	1	187	3	1	99
side salad	1	42	3	1	48
SALAD DRESSINGS					
bleu cheese	½ pkg	16	17	3	171
French	½ pkg	<1	10	2	114
house	½ pkg	7	17	3	163
lite vinaigrette	½ pkg	1	1	tr	25
Oriental	½ pkg	1	2	tr	51
Thousand Island	½ pkg	24	20	3	198
SHAKES					
chocolate	1	30	9	4	383
strawberry	1	32	9	4	362
vanilla	1	31	8	4	352
SIDE DISHES					
french fries	1 regular serving	9	12	5	220
Roy Rogers					
BEVERAGES					
hot chocolate	1	35	2	?	123
BREAKFAST ITEMS					
crescent roll	1	<5	18	?	287
crescent sandwich	1	148	27	?	401
w/bacon	1	156	30	?	431
w/ham	1	189	42	?	557
w/sausage	1	168	29	?	449

	Portion	Chol (mg)	Total Fat (g)	Satur'd Fat (g)	Total Calor
egg & biscuit platter	1	284	27	?	394
w/bacon	1	294	30	?	435
w/ham	1	304	29	?	442
w/sausage	1	325	41	?	550
pancake platter, w/syrup & butter	1	53	15	?	452
w/bacon	1	63	18	?	493
w/ham	1	73	17	?	506
w/sausage	1	94	30	?	608
BURGERS & SANDWICHES					
bacon cheeseburger	1	103	39	?	581
cheeseburger	1	95	37	?	563
hamburger	1	73	28	?	456
roast beef					
regular	1	55	10	?	317
w/cheese	1	77	19	?	424
large	1	73	12	?	360
w/cheese	1	95	21	?	467
RR Bar Burger	1	115	39	?	611
CHICKEN					
breast	1	118	24	?	412
breast & wing	1 each	165	37	24	604
drumstick/leg	1	40	8	24	140
nuggets	6	51	17	24	267
thigh	1	85	20	24	296
thigh & leg	1 each	125	28	24	436
wing	1	47	13	24	192
DESSERTS					
brownie	1	10	11	?	264
danish					
apple	1	15	12	?	249
cheese	1	11	12	?	254
cherry	1	11	14	?	271
strawberry shortcake	1 serving	28	19	?	447
sundaes					
caramel	1	23	9	?	293
hot fudge	1	23	13	?	337
strawberry	1	23	7	?	216
SALAD BAR ITEMS					
bacon bits	1 T	?	?	?	33
beets, sliced	¼ c	?	0	?	16
broccoli	½ c	?	0	?	20
carrots, shredded	¼ c	?	?	?	42
cheddar cheese	¼ c	?	9	?	112
Chinese noodles	¼ c	?	3	?	55
croutons	2 T	?	?	?	70
cucumbers	5–6 slices	?	0	?	4

	Portion	Chol (mg)	Total Fat (g)	Satur'd Fat (g)	Total Calor
eggs, chopped	2 T	?	4	?	55
green peas	¼ c	?	0	?	7
green peppers	¼ c	?	0	?	4
lettuce	1 c	?	0	?	10
macaroni salad	2 T	?	4	?	60
mushrooms	¼ c	?	0	?	5
potato salad	2 T	?	3	?	50
sunflower seeds	2 T	?	13	?	157
tomatoes	3 slices	?	0	?	20

SALAD DRESSINGS

bacon & tomato	2 T	?	12	?	136
bleu cheese	2 T	?	16	?	150
low-cal Italian	2 T	?	6	?	70
Ranch	2 T	?	14	?	155
Thousand Island	2 T	?	16	?	160

SHAKES

chocolate	1	37	10	?	358
strawberry	1	37	10	?	315
vanilla	1	40	11	?	306

SIDE DISHES

biscuit	1	<5	12	?	231
cole slaw	1 serving	<5	7	?	110
french fries	1 regular serving	42	14	?	268
	1 large serving	56	18	?	357
hot topped potato					
plain	1	0	tr	?	211
w/bacon & cheese	1	34	22	?	397
w/broccoli & cheese	1	<19	18	?	376
w/oleo	1	0	7	?	274
w/sour cream & chives	1	31	21	?	408
w/taco beef & cheese	1	37	22	?	463
macaroni	1 serving	<5	11	?	186
potato salad	1 serving	<5	6	?	107

Wendy's
BEVERAGES

hot chocolate	1	tr	1	?	110
lemonade	1	0	<1	?	160

BREAKFAST ITEMS

bacon	1 strip	5	2	?	30
breakfast sandwich	1	200	19	?	370
buttermilk biscuit	1	tr	17	?	320
danish					
apple	1	?	14	?	360
cheese	1	?	21	?	430
cinnamon raisin	1	?	18	?	410

	Portion	Chol (mg)	Total Fat (g)	Satur'd Fat (g)	Total Calor
French toast	2 slices	115	19	?	400
French toast toppings					
apple	1 pkt	0	<1	?	130
blueberry	1 pkt	0	<1	?	60
fried egg	1	230	6	?	90
grape jelly	1 pkt	0	<1	?	40
omelet #1: ham & cheese	1	355	21	?	290
omelet #2: ham, cheese, & mushroom	1	450	17	?	250
omelet #3: ham, cheese, onion, & green pepper	1	525	19	?	280
omelet #4: mushroom, green pepper, & onion	1	460	15	?	210
potatoes	1 serving	20	22	?	360
sausage gravy	6 oz	85	36	?	440
sausage patty	1	45	18	?	200
scrambled eggs	2 eggs	450	12	?	190
strawberry jam	1 pkt	0	<1	?	40
syrup	1 pkt	0	<1	?	140
toast, w/margarine					
wheat	2 slices	5	8	?	190
white	2 slices	20	9	?	250

BURGER & SANDWICH COMPONENTS

	Portion	Chol (mg)	Total Fat (g)	Satur'd Fat (g)	Total Calor
American cheese slice	1	15	6	?	60
bacon	1 strip	5	2	?	30
buns					
kaiser	1	5	2	?	180
multigrain	1	tr	3	?	140
white	1	tr	2	?	140
catsup	1 t	0	<1	?	6
hamburger patty, ¼ lb	1	75	14	?	210
lettuce	1 leaf	0	<1	?	2
mayonnaise	1 T	10	10	?	90
mustard	1 t	0	<1	?	4
onion	3 rings	0	<1	?	2
pickles, dill	4 slices	0	<1	?	2
taco sauce	1 pkt	0	<1	?	10
tartar sauce	1 T	?	9	?	80
tomatoes	1 slice	0	<1	?	2

BURGERS & SANDWICHES

	Portion	Chol (mg)	Total Fat (g)	Satur'd Fat (g)	Total Calor
Big Classic (two ¼-lb hamburger patties, mayonnaise, catsup, pickles, onion, tomatoes, lettuce, kaiser bun)	1	80	25	?	470
chicken breast fillet	1	60	10	?	200
chicken fried steak	1	95	41	?	580

	Portion	Chol (mg)	Total Fat (g)	Satur'd Fat (g)	Total Calor
fish fillet	1	45	11	?	210
Kids' Meal Hamburger	1	35	9	?	200

CHICKEN NUGGETS & SAUCES

Crispy Nuggets					
cooked in animal/vegetable oil	6	55	21	?	290
cooked in vegetable oil	6	50	21	?	310
barbecue sauce	1 pkt	0	<1	?	50
honey	1 pkt	0	<1	?	45
sweet & sour sauce	1 pkt	0	<1	?	45
sweet mustard sauce	1 pkt	0	1	?	50

CHILI

chili	1 regular serving	75	8	?	240

CONDIMENTS, SAUCES, & MISCELLANEOUS ITEMS

catsup	1 pkt	0	<1	?	12
cheese sauce	2 oz	20	12	?	140
half & half	⅜ oz	5	1	?	14
hot chili seasoning	1 pkt	?	<1	?	6
margarine					
liquid	½ oz	0	11	?	100
whipped	1 T	0	8	?	70
nondairy creamer	⅜ oz	0	1	?	14
saltines	2	?	<1	?	25
sour cream	2 t	5	2	?	20
sugar	1 pkt	0	0	?	14

DESSERTS

chocolate chip cookie	1	5	17	?	320
Frosty dairy dessert	1 regular serving	50	14	?	400

SALAD BAR ITEMS

alfalfa sprouts	1 oz	0	<1	?	8
American cheese	1 oz	5	7	?	90
bacon bits	⅛ oz	tr	<1	?	10
blueberries	1 T	0	<1	?	6
bread sticks	2	0	1	?	35
broccoli	½ c	0	<1	?	12
cabbage, red	¼ c	0	<1	?	4
cantaloupe	2 pieces	0	<1	?	18
carrots	¼ c	0	<1	?	10
cauliflower	½ c	0	<1	?	12
celery	1 T	0	<1	?	0
cheddar cheese	1 oz	tr	6	?	80
cherry peppers	1 T	0	<1	?	6
chow mein noodles	½ oz	?	4	?	70
cole slaw	¼ c	40	5	?	80

	Portion	Chol (mg)	Total Fat (g)	Satur'd Fat (g)	Total Calor
cottage cheese	½ c	20	4	?	110
croutons	½ oz	?	3	?	60
cucumbers	4 slices	0	<1	?	2
eggs	1 T	90	2	?	30
grapefruit	2 oz	0	<1	?	10
grapes	¼ c	0	<1	?	30
green peas	1 oz	0	<1	?	25
green peppers	¼ c	0	<1	?	8
honeydew melon	2 pieces	0	<1	?	20
jalapeño peppers	1 T	0	<1	?	9
lettuce					
iceberg	1 c	0	<1	?	8
romaine	1 c	0	<1	?	10
mozzarella cheese	1 oz	tr	7	?	90
mushrooms	¼ c	0	<1	?	4
oranges	2 oz	0	<1	?	25
Parmesan cheese, grated	1 oz	20	9	?	130
pasta salad	¼ c	5	6	?	130
peaches	2 slices	0	<1	?	17
pepper rings	1 T	0	<1	?	2
pineapple chunks	½ c	0	<1	?	70
provolone cheese	1 oz	tr	7	?	90
radishes	½ oz	0	<1	?	2
red onions	3 rings	0	<1	?	2
strawberries	2 oz	0	<1	?	18
sunflower seeds & raisins	1 oz	0	10	?	140
Swiss cheese	1 oz	5	7	?	90
tomatoes	1 oz	0	<1	?	6
turkey ham	¼ c	?	2	?	50
watermelon	2 pieces	0	<1	?	18

SALAD DRESSINGS

Regular

bleu cheese	1 T	10	7	?	60
celery seed	1 T	5	6	?	70
French style	1 T	0	5	?	70
Golden Italian	1 T	0	4	?	50
oil	1 T	0	14	?	120
Ranch	1 T	5	6	?	50
Thousand Island	1 T	10	7	?	70
wine vinegar	1 T	0	<1	?	2

Reduced-Calorie

bacon/tomato	1 T	tr	4	?	45
creamy cucumber	1 T	tr	5	?	50
Italian	1 T	0	2	?	25
Thousand Island	1 T	5	4	?	45

	Portion	Chol (mg)	Total Fat (g)	Satur'd Fat (g)	Total Calor
SIDE DISHES					
french fries					
cooked in animal/vegetable oil	1 regular serving	15	15	?	310
cooked in vegetable oil	1 regular serving	5	15	?	300
hot stuffed baked potatoes					
plain	1	tr	2	?	250
bacon & cheese	1	22	30	?	570
broccoli & cheese	1	22	25	?	500
cheese	1	22	34	?	590
chili & cheese	1	22	20	?	510
sour cream & chives	1	15	24	?	460
TACO SALAD					
taco salad	1 serving	45	19	?	430
taco sauce	1 pkt	0	<1	?	10

❑ FATS, OILS, & SHORTENINGS
See also BUTTER & MARGARINE SPREADS

Fats

	Portion	Chol (mg)	Total Fat (g)	Satur'd Fat (g)	Total Calor
beef tallow	1 c	223	205	102	1,849
	1 T	14	13	6	116
butter oil, anhydrous	1 c	524	204	127	1,795
	1 T	33	13	8	112
chicken fat	1 T	11	13	4	115
duck fat	1 T	13	13	4	115
goose fat	1 T	13	13	4	115
lard (pork)	1 c	195	205	80	1,849
	1 T	12	13	5	116

Oils

	Portion	Chol (mg)	Total Fat (g)	Satur'd Fat (g)	Total Calor
almond	1 c	0	218	18	1,927
	1 T	0	14	1	120
apricot kernel	1 T	0	14	1	120
babassu	1 T	0	14	11	120
cocoa butter	1 c	0	218	130	1,927
	1 T	0	14	8	120
coconut	1 c	0	218	189	1,927
	1 T	0	14	12	120
corn	1 c	0	218	28	1,927
	1 T	0	14	2	120
cottonseed	1 c	0	218	56	1,927
	1 T	0	14	4	120

	Portion	Chol (mg)	Total Fat (g)	Satur'd Fat (g)	Total Calor
cupu assu	1 T	0	14	7	120
grapeseed	1 T	0	14	1	120
hazelnut	1 c	0	218	16	1,927
	1 T	0	14	1	120
linseed	1 T	0	14	1	120
nutmeg butter	1 T	0	14	12	120
olive	1 c	0	216	29	1,909
	1 T	0	14	2	119
palm	1 c	0	218	107	1,927
	1 T	0	14	7	120
palm kernel	1 T	0	14	11	120
peanut	1 c	0	216	36	1,909
	1 T	0	14	2	119
poppy seed	1 T	0	14	2	120
rapeseed, no erucic acid content	1 T	0	14	1	120
rice bran	1 T	0	14	3	120
safflower					
linoleic (over 70%)	1 c	0	218	20	1,927
	1 T	0	14	1	120
oleic (over 70%)	1 c	0	218	13	1,927
	1 T	0	14	1	120
sesame	1 c	0	218	31	1,927
	1 T	0	14	2	120
sheanut	1 T	0	14	6	120
soybean	1 c	0	218	31	1,927
	1 T	0	14	2	120
soybean (hydrogenated)	1 c	0	218	33	1,927
	1 T	0	14	2	120
soybean (hydrogenated) & cottonseed	1 c	0	218	39	1,927
	1 T	0	14	2	120
soybean lecithin (values for commercial products containing 70% soybean phosphatide in 30% soybean oil)	1 c	0	218	33	1,927
	1 T	0	14	2	120
sunflower					
hydrogenated	1 c	0	218	28	1,927
	1 T	0	14	2	120
linoleic (<60%)	1 c	0	218	22	1,927
	1 T	0	14	1	120
teaseed	1 T	0	14	3	120
tomato seed	1 T	0	14	3	120
ucuhuba butter	1 T	0	14	12	120
walnut	1 c	0	218	20	1,927
	1 T	0	14	1	120
wheat germ	1 T	0	14	3	120

	Portion	Chol (mg)	Total Fat (g)	Satur'd Fat (g)	Total Calor
Shortenings					
HOUSEHOLD					
lard & vegetable oil	1 c	?	205	83	1,845
	1 T	?	13	5	115
soybean (hydrogenated) & cottonseed (hydrogenated)	1 c	?	205	51	1,812
	1 T	?	13	3	113
soybean (hydrogenated) & palm	1 c	0	205	63	1,812
	1 T	0	13	4	113
INDUSTRIAL					
lard & vegetable oil	1 c	?	205	73	1,845
	1 T	?	13	5	115
soybean (hydrogenated) & cottonseed	1 c	0	205	53	1,812
	1 T	0	13	3	113
SPECIAL FOR BREAD					
soybean (hydrogenated) & cottonseed	1 c	0	205	45	1,812
	1 T	0	13	3	113
SPECIAL FOR CAKE MIX					
soybean (hydrogenated) & cottonseed (hydrogenated)	1 c	0	205	56	1,812
	1 T	0	13	4	113
SPECIAL FOR CONFECTIONERY					
coconut (hydrogenated) &/or palm kernel (hydrogenated)	1 c	0	205	187	1,812
	1 T	0	13	12	113
fractionated palm	1 c	0	218	143	1,927
	1 T	0	14	9	120
SPECIAL FOR FRYING					
Regular					
soybean (hydrogenated) & cottonseed (hydrogenated)	1 c	0	205	32	1,812
	1 T	0	13	2	113
Heavy Duty					
beef tallow & cottonseed	1 c	?	205	92	1,845
	1 T	?	13	6	115
palm (hydrogenated)	1 c	10	205	97	1,812
	1 T	0	13	6	113
soybean (hydrogenated) linoleic (<1%)	1 c	0	205	43	1,812
	1 T	0	13	3	113
linoleic (about 30%), stabilized w/silicones	1 c	0	205	38	1,812
	1 T	0	13	2	113

	Portion	Chol (mg)	Total Fat (g)	Satur'd Fat (g)	Total Calor
■ BRAND NAME					
Arrowhead Mills					
corn germ oil, unrefined	1 T	0	14	2	120
olive oil, unrefined	1 T	0	14	1	120
safflower oil, unrefined	1 T	0	14	2	120
sesame oil, unrefined	1 T	0	14	2	120
Mazola					
corn oil	1 T	0	14	2	120
No-Stick	2½-second spray	0	1	tr	6
Planters					
peanut oil	1 T	0	14	2	120
Rokeach					
Neutral Nyafat	1 T	?	11	?	99

□ FISH *See* SEAFOOD & SEAFOOD PRODUCTS

□ FLOURS & CORNMEALS
See also NUTS & NUT-BASED BUTTERS, FLOURS, MEALS, MILKS, PASTES, & POWDERS; SEEDS & SEED-BASED BUTTERS, FLOURS, & MEALS

	Portion	Chol (mg)	Total Fat (g)	Satur'd Fat (g)	Total Calor
arrowroot flour	1 T	0	0	?	29
barley flour	1 T	0	tr	?	28
	1 c	0	2	?	401
buckwheat flour					
dark	1 oz	0	1	?	92
light	1 c	0	1	tr	340
carob flour	1 T	0	tr	tr	14
	1 c	0	1	tr	185
corn flour, sifted	1 c	0	3	?	405
masa harina	⅓ c	0	2	?	137
masa trigo	⅓ c	0	4	?	149
white, tortilla, lime-treated	1 oz	0	2	?	103
yellow, tortilla, untreated	1 oz	0	1	?	101
corn germ, toasted	1 oz	0	7	?	130
cornmeal					
whole-ground, dry					
bolted	1 c	0	4	1	122
unbolted	1 c	0	5	1	122
degermed, enriched					
dry	1 c	0	2	tr	138
cooked	1 c	0	tr	tr	240

	Portion	Chol (mg)	Total Fat (g)	Satur'd Fat (g)	Total Calor
cornmeal *(cont.)*					
white, self-rising, dry	1 oz or ⅙ c	0	1	?	98
cornstarch	1 T	0	tr	?	35
manioc (casava) flour	3½ oz	0	1	?	320
potato flour	1 c	0	1	tr	628
rice bran	1 oz	0	tr	?	80
rice flour	1 c	0	tr	?	479
rice polish	1 oz	0	2	?	101
rye flour					
dark	3½ oz	0	3	?	327
light	3½ oz	0	1	?	357
rye wheat flour	1 c	0	1	?	400
soy flour *See* SOYBEANS & SOYBEAN PRODUCTS					
wheat & gluten flour	1 c	0	3	?	529
wheat flour, enriched					
all-purpose					
sifted	1 c	0	1	tr	420
unsifted	1 c	0	1	tr	455
bread, sifted	1 c	0	1	?	409
cake or pastry, sifted	1 c	0	1	tr	350
self-rising, unsifted	1 c	0	1	tr	440
whole-wheat & soy flour	3½ oz	0	7	?	365
whole-wheat flour, from hard wheats	1 c	0	2	tr	400
whole-wheat flour, straight, soft	3½ oz	0	1	?	364

- **BRAND NAME**

Argo

Argo & Kingsford's Corn Starch	1 T	0	0	0	30

Arrowhead Mills

barley flour	2 oz	0	1	?	200
brown rice flour	2 oz	0	1	?	200
buckwheat flour	2 oz	0	1	?	190
corn flour, yellow	2 oz	0	2	?	210
cornmeal					
blue	2 oz	0	3	?	210
hi-lysine	2 oz	0	2	?	210
yellow	2 oz	0	2	?	210
Ezekiel flour	2 oz	0	1	?	200
garbanzo flour	2 oz	0	3	?	200
millet flour	2 oz	0	2	?	185
oat flour	2 oz	0	1	?	200
pastry flour	2 oz	0	1	?	180
rye flour	2 oz	0	1	?	190
triticale flour	2 oz	0	1	?	190
unbleached white flour	2 oz	0	1	?	200

	Portion	Chol (mg)	Total Fat (g)	Satur'd Fat (g)	Total Calor
vital wheat gluten	1 oz	0	1	?	100
whole-wheat flour	2 oz	0	1	?	200
Aunt Jemima					
CORNMEAL					
bolted white, mix	⅙ c	0	1	?	99
bolted yellow, mix	⅙ c	0	tr	?	97
buttermilk self-rising white, mix	3 T	0	1	?	101
enriched white	3 T	0	1	?	102
enriched yellow	3 T	0	1	?	102
self-rising white	⅙ c	0	1	?	98
self-rising white enriched bolted	⅙ c	0	1	?	99
FLOUR					
enriched self-rising	¼ c	?	tr	?	109
Fearn					
rice flour	½ c	0	0	tr	270
Featherweight					
potato starch	1 c	?	1	?	620
rice flour	1 c	?	1	?	500
Heckers					
flour	about 1 c or 4 oz	0	1	?	380–400
Quaker Oats					
masa harina de maiz	⅓ c	?	2	?	137
masa trigo	⅓ c	?	4	?	149

❑ FRANKFURTERS *See* PROCESSED MEAT & POULTRY PRODUCTS

❑ FRUIT, FRESH & PROCESSED
See also PICKLES, OLIVES, RELISHES, & CHUTNEYS; SNACKS

acerolas, raw	1 c	0	tr	?	31
apples					
raw					
w/skin	1 fruit = 4.9 oz	0	tr	tr	81
w/out skin	1 fruit = 4½ oz	0	tr	tr	72
baked in microwave, w/out skin	½ c sliced	0	tr	tr	48

	Portion	Chol (mg)	Total Fat (g)	Satur'd Fat (g)	Total Calor
apples *(cont.)*					
boiled, w/out skin	1½ c sliced	0	tr	tr	46
canned, sweetened, unheated	½ c sliced	0	1	tr	68
dehydrated, sulfured					
cooked	½ c	0	tr	tr	71
uncooked	½ c	0	tr	tr	104
dried, sulfured					
cooked, w/added sugar	½ c	0	tr	tr	116
cooked, w/out added sugar	½ c	0	tr	tr	72
uncooked	2¼ oz	0	tr	tr	155
	1 c	0	tr	tr	209
frozen, unsweetened					
heated	½ c sliced	0	tr	tr	48
unheated	½ c sliced	0	tr	tr	41
applesauce, canned					
sweetened	½ c	0	tr	tr	97
unsweetened	½ c	0	tr	tr	53
apricots					
raw	3 fruit = 3.7 oz	0	tr	tr	51
canned, w/skin					
in water	3 halves + 1¾ T liquid	0	tr	tr	22
in juice	3 halves + 1¾ T liquid	0	tr	tr	40
in extra light syrup	3 halves + 1¾ T liquid	0	tr	tr	41
in light syrup	3 halves + 1¾ T liquid	0	tr	tr	54
in heavy syrup	3 halves + 1¾ T liquid	0	tr	tr	70
canned, w/out skin					
in water	2 fruit + 2 T liquid	0	tr	tr	20
in heavy syrup	2 fruit + 2 T liquid	0	tr	tr	75
in extra heavy syrup	2 fruit + 2 T liquid	0	tr	tr	87
dehydrated (low-moisture), sulfured					
cooked	½ c	0	tr	tr	156
uncooked	½ c	0	tr	tr	192
dried, sulfured					
cooked, w/added sugar	½ c halves	0	tr	tr	153

	Portion	Chol (mg)	Total Fat (g)	Satur'd Fat (g)	Total Calor
cooked, w/out added sugar	½ c halves	0	tr	tr	106
uncooked	10 halves	0	tr	tr	83
frozen, sweetened	½ c	0	tr	tr	119
avocados, raw					
all commercial varieties	1 fruit = 7.1 oz	0	31	5	324
	1 c puree	0	35	6	370
California	1 fruit = 6.1 oz	0	30	4	306
	1 c puree	0	40	6	407
Florida	1 fruit = 10.7 oz	0	27	5	339
	1 c puree	0	20	4	257
bananas					
raw	1 fruit = 4 oz	0	tr	1	105
dehydrated (banana powder)	1 T	0	tr	tr	21
blackberries					
raw	½ c	0	tr	?	37
canned, in heavy syrup	½ c	0	tr	?	118
frozen, unsweetened	1 c	0	1	?	97
blueberries					
raw	1 c	0	1	?	82
canned, in heavy syrup	½ c	0	tr	?	112
frozen					
sweetened	1 c	0	tr	?	187
unsweetened	1 c	0	1	?	78
boysenberries					
canned, in heavy syrup	½ c	0	tr	?	113
frozen, unsweetened	1 c	0	tr	?	66
breadfruit, raw	¼ small fruit = 3.4 oz	0	tr	?	99
candied fruit See BAKING INGREDIENTS					
cantaloupe See melons, below					
carambolas, raw	1 fruit = 4½ oz	0	tr	?	42
carissa plums, raw	1 fruit = 0.7 oz	0	tr	?	12
casaba See melons, below					
cherimoyas, raw	1 fruit = 19¼ oz	0	2	?	515
cherries, sour, red					
raw	1 c w/pits	0	tr	tr	51
canned					
in water	½ c	0	tr	tr	43
in light syrup	½ c	0	tr	tr	94
in heavy syrup	½ c	0	tr	tr	116
in extra heavy syrup	½ c	0	tr	tr	148

	Portion	Chol (mg)	Total Fat (g)	Satur'd Fat (g)	Total Calor
cherries, sour, red *(cont.)*					
frozen, unsweetened	1 c	0	1	tr	72
cherries, sweet					
raw	10 fruit = 2.4 oz	0	1	tr	49
canned					
in water	½ c	0	tr	tr	57
in juice	½ c	0	tr	tr	68
in light syrup	½ c	0	tr	tr	85
in heavy syrup	½ c	0	tr	tr	107
in extra heavy syrup	½ c	0	tr	tr	133
frozen, sweetened	1 c	0	tr	tr	232
Chinese gooseberries *See* kiwi fruit, *below*					
coconut *See* BAKING INGREDIENTS; NUTS & NUT-BASED BUTTERS, FLOURS, MEALS, MILKS, PASTES, & POWDERS					
crabapples, raw	1 c sliced	0	tr	tr	83
cranberries, raw	1 c whole	0	tr	?	46
cranberry sauce, canned, sweetened	½ c	0	tr	?	209
currants					
European, black, raw	½ c	0	tr	tr	36
red & white, raw	½ c	0	tr	tr	31
zante, dried	½ c	0	tr	tr	204
custard apples, raw	edible portion = 3½ oz	0	1	?	101
dates, domestic, dry	10 fruit = 2.9 oz	0	tr	?	228
elderberries, raw	1 c	0	1	?	105
figs					
raw	1 medium fruit = 1¾ oz	0	tr	tr	37
canned					
in water	3 fruit + 1¾ T liquid	0	tr	tr	42
in light syrup	3 fruit + 1¾ T liquid	0	tr	tr	58
in heavy syrup	3 fruit + 1¾ T liquid	0	tr	tr	75
in extra heavy syrup	3 fruit + 1¾ T liquid	0	tr	tr	91
dried					
cooked	½ c	0	1	tr	140
uncooked	10 fruit = 6.6 oz	0	2	tr	477
fruit cocktail, canned					
in water	½ c	0	tr	tr	40

	Portion	Chol (mg)	Total Fat (g)	Satur'd Fat (g)	Total Calor
in juice	½ c	0	tr	tr	56
in extra light syrup	½ c	0	tr	tr	55
in light syrup	½ c	0	tr	tr	72
in heavy syrup	½ c	0	tr	tr	93
in extra heavy syrup	½ c	0	tr	tr	115
fruit salad, canned					
in water	½ c	0	tr	tr	37
in juice	½ c	0	tr	tr	62
in light syrup	½ c	0	tr	tr	73
in heavy syrup	½ c	0	tr	tr	94
in extra heavy syrup	½ c	0	tr	tr	114
fruit salad, tropical, canned, in heavy syrup	½ c	0	tr	?	110
gooseberries					
raw	1 c	0	1	tr	67
canned, in light syrup	½ c	0	tr	tr	93
grandillas *See* passion fruit, *below*					
grapefruit					
raw, pink & red	½ fruit = 4.3 oz	0	tr	tr	37
raw, white	½ fruit = 4.2 oz	0	tr	tr	39
canned					
in water	½ c	0	tr	tr	44
in juice	½ c	0	tr	tr	46
in light syrup	½ c	0	tr	tr	76
grapes					
American type, raw	10 fruit = 0.8 oz	0	tr	tr	15
European type, raw	10 fruit = 1.8 oz	0	tr	tr	36
Thompson seedless, canned					
in water	½ c	0	tr	tr	48
in heavy syrup, solids & liquids	½ c	0	tr	tr	94
groundcherries, raw	½ c	0	tr	?	37
guavas					
common, raw	1 fruit = 3.2 oz	0	1	tr	45
strawberry, raw	1 fruit = 0.2 oz	0	tr	tr	4
guava sauce, cooked	½ c	0	tr	tr	43
honeydew *See* melons, *below*					
jackfruit, raw	edible portion = 3½ oz	0	tr	tr	94
jujubes					
raw	edible portion = 3½ oz	0	tr	?	79

	Portion	Chol (mg)	Total Fat (g)	Satur'd Fat (g)	Total Calor
jujubes *(cont.)*					
dried	edible portion = 3½ oz	0	1	?	287
kiwi fruit, raw	1 medium fruit = 2.7 oz	0	tr	?	46
kumquats, raw	1 fruit = 0.7 oz	0	tr	?	12
lemon peel, raw	1 t	0	tr	tr	?
	1 T	0	tr	tr	?
lemons, raw					
w/peel	1 medium fruit = 3.8 oz	0	tr	tr	22
w/out peel	1 medium fruit = 2 oz	0	tr	tr	17
limes, raw	1 fruit = 2.4 oz	0	tr	tr	20
litchis *See* lychees, *below*					
loganberries, frozen	1 c	0	tr	?	80
longans					
raw	1 fruit = 0.1 oz	0	0	?	2
dried	edible portion = 3½ oz	0	tr	?	286
loquats, raw	1 fruit = 0.3 oz	0	tr	tr	5
lychees					
raw	1 fruit = 0.3 oz	0	tr	?	6
dried	edible portion = 3½ oz	0	1	?	277
mammy apples, raw	1 fruit = 29.8 oz	0	4	?	431
mangos, raw	1 fruit = 7.3 oz	0	1	tr	135
melon balls, frozen, cantaloupe & honeydew	1 c	0	tr	?	55
melons					
cantaloupe, raw	½ fruit = 9.4 oz	22	1	?	94
	1 c cubed	13	tr	?	57
casaba, raw	1/10 fruit = 5.8 oz	0	tr	?	43
	1 c cubed	0	tr	?	45
honeydew, raw	1/10 fruit = 4½ oz	0	tr	?	46
	1 c cubed	0	tr	?	60

	Portion	Chol (mg)	Total Fat (g)	Satur'd Fat (g)	Total Calor
muskmelons *See* melons: cantaloupe, *above*					
mixed fruit					
canned, in heavy syrup, solids & liquids	½ c	0	tr	tr	92
dried	11 oz	0	1	tr	712
frozen, sweetened	1 c	0	tr	tr	245
mulberries, raw	10 fruit = ½ oz	0	tr	?	7
muskmelons *See* melons: cantaloupe, *above*					
natal plums *See* carissa plums, *above*					
nectarines, raw	1 fruit = 4.8 oz	0	1	?	67
oheloberries, raw	10 fruit = 0.4 oz	0	tr	?	3
orange peel, raw	1 t	0	0	0	?
	1 T	0	tr	tr	?
oranges, raw					
w/peel	1 fruit = 5.6 oz	0	tr	tr	64
w/out peel					
all commercial varieties	1 fruit = 4.6 oz	0	tr	tr	62
California, navels	1 fruit = 4.9 oz	0	tr	tr	65
California, Valencias	1 fruit = 4.3 oz	0	tr	tr	59
Florida	1 fruit = 5.3 oz	0	tr	tr	69
papayas, raw	1 fruit = 10.7 oz	0	tr	tr	117
passion fruit, purple, raw	1 fruit = 0.6 oz	0	tr	?	18
peaches					
raw	1 fruit = 3.1 oz	0	tr	tr	37
canned, clingstone					
in water	1 half + 1⅔ T liquid	0	tr	tr	18
in extra light syrup	1 half + 1⅔ T liquid	0	tr	tr	32
in light syrup	1 half + 1¾ T liquid	0	tr	tr	44
canned, clingstone & freestone					
in juice	1 half + 1⅔ T liquid	0	tr	tr	34

	Portion	Chol (mg)	Total Fat (g)	Satur'd Fat (g)	Total Calor
peaches: canned *(cont.)*					
in heavy syrup	1 half + 1¾ T liquid	0	tr	tr	60
canned, freestone in extra heavy syrup	1 half + 1¾ T liquid	0	tr	tr	77
dehydrated (low-moisture), sulfured					
cooked	½ c	0	1	tr	161
uncooked	½ c	0	1	tr	188
dried, sulfured					
cooked, w/added sugar	½ c halves	0	tr	tr	139
cooked, w/out added sugar	½ c halves	0	tr	tr	99
uncooked	10 halves	0	1	tr	311
frozen, sweetened	1 c sliced, thawed	0	tr	tr	235
peaches, spiced, canned, in heavy syrup	1 fruit + 2 T liquid	0	tr	tr	66
pears					
raw	1 fruit = 5.8 oz	0	1	tr	98
canned					
in water	1 half + 1⅔ T liquid	0	tr	tr	22
in juice	1 half + 1⅔ T liquid	0	tr	tr	38
in extra light syrup	1 half + 1⅔ T liquid	0	tr	tr	36
in light syrup	1 half + 1¾ T liquid	0	tr	tr	45
in heavy syrup	1 half + 1¾ T liquid	0	tr	tr	58
in extra heavy syrup	1 half + 1¾ T liquid	0	tr	tr	77
dried, sulfured					
cooked, w/added sugar	½ c halves	0	tr	tr	196
cooked, w/out added sugar	½ c halves	0	tr	tr	163
uncooked	10 halves	0	1	tr	459
persimmons					
Japanese					
raw	1 fruit = 5.9 oz	0	tr	?	118

	Portion	Chol (mg)	Total Fat (g)	Satur'd Fat (g)	Total Calor
dried	1 fruit = 1.2 oz	0	tr	?	93
native, raw	1 fruit = 0.9 oz	0	tr	?	32
pineapple					
raw	1 slice = 3 oz	0	tr	tr	42
	1 c diced	0	1	tr	77
canned					
in water	1 slice + 1¼ T liquid	0	tr	tr	19
	1 c tidbits	0	tr	tr	79
in juice	1 slice + 1¼ T liquid	0	tr	tr	35
	1 c chunks or tidbits	0	tr	tr	150
in light syrup	1 slice + 1¼ T liquid	0	tr	tr	30
	1 c	0	tr	tr	131
in heavy syrup	1 slice + 1¼ T liquid	0	tr	tr	45
	1 c chunks, tidbits, or crushed	0	tr	tr	199
in extra heavy syrup	1 slice + 1¼ T liquid	0	tr	tr	48
	1 c chunks or crushed	0	tr	tr	217
frozen, sweetened	½ c chunks	0	tr	tr	104
pitangas, raw	1 fruit = 0.2 oz	0	tr	?	2
	1 c	0	1	?	57
plantains					
raw	1 fruit = 6.3 oz	0	1	?	218
cooked	½ c sliced	0	tr	?	89
plums, purple					
raw	1 fruit = 2.3 oz	0	tr	tr	36
canned					
in water	3 fruit + 2 T liquid	0	tr	tr	39
	1 c	0	tr	tr	102

	Portion	Chol (mg)	Total Fat (g)	Satur'd Fat (g)	Total Calor
plums: canned *(cont.)*					
in juice	3 fruit + 2 T liquid	0	tr	tr	55
	1 c	0	tr	tr	146
in light syrup	3 fruit + 2¾ T liquid	0	tr	tr	83
	1 c	0	tr	tr	158
in heavy syrup	3 fruit + 2¾ T liquid	0	tr	tr	119
	1 c	0	tr	tr	230
in extra heavy syrup	3 fruit + 2¾ T liquid	0	tr	tr	135
	1 c	0	tr	tr	265
pomegranates, raw	1 fruit = 5.4 oz	0	tr	?	104
prickly pears, raw	1 fruit = 3.6 oz	0	1	?	42
prunes					
canned, in heavy syrup	5 fruit + 2 T liquid	0	tr	tr	90
	1 c	0	tr	tr	245
dehydrated (low-moisture)					
cooked	½ c	0	tr	tr	158
uncooked	½ c	0	tr	tr	224
dried					
cooked, w/added sugar	½ c	0	tr	tr	147
cooked, w/out added sugar	½ c	0	tr	tr	113
uncooked	10 fruit = 3 oz	0	tr	tr	201
	1 c	0	1	tr	385
pummelos, raw	1 fruit = 21.4 oz	0	tr	?	228
	1 c sections	0	tr	?	71
quinces, raw	1 fruit = 3.2 oz	0	tr	tr	53
raisins					
golden seedless	1 c not packed	0	1	tr	437
	1 c packed	0	1	tr	498
seeded	1 c not packed	0	1	tr	428
	1 c packed	0	1	tr	488
seedless	1 c not packed	0	1	tr	434
	1 c packed	0	1	tr	494

	Portion	Chol (mg)	Total Fat (g)	Satur'd Fat (g)	Total Calor
raspberries, red					
raw	1 c	0	1	tr	61
canned, in heavy syrup, solids & liquids	½ c	0	tr	tr	117
frozen, sweetened	1 c	0	tr	tr	256
	10 oz pkg	0	tr	tr	291
rhubarb					
raw	½ c diced	0	tr	?	13
frozen					
cooked, w/added sugar	½ c	0	tr	?	139
uncooked	½ c	0	tr	?	14
rose apples, raw	edible portion = 3½ oz	0	tr	?	25
roselles, raw	1 c	0	tr	?	28
sapodillas, raw	1 fruit = 6 oz	0	2	?	140
sapotes, raw	1 fruit = 7.9 oz	0	1	?	301
soursops, raw	1 fruit = 22 oz	0	2	?	416
starfruit *See* carambolas, *above*					
strawberries					
raw	1 c	0	1	tr	45
canned, in heavy syrup	½ c	0	tr	tr	117
frozen, sweetened					
sliced	1 c	0	tr	tr	245
	10 oz pkg	0	tr	tr	273
whole	1 c	0	tr	tr	200
	10 oz pkg	0	tr	tr	223
frozen, unsweetened	1 c	0	tr	tr	52
sugar apples, raw	1 fruit = 5½ oz	0	tr	?	146
Surinam cherries *See* pitangas, *above*					
sweetsops *See* sugar apples, *above*					
tamarinds, raw	1 fruit = 0.1 oz	0	tr	tr	5
tangerines					
raw	1 fruit = 3 oz	0	tr	tr	37
canned					
in juice, solids & liquids	½ c	0	tr	tr	46
in light syrup, solids & liquids	½ c	0	tr	tr	76
watermelon, raw	¹⁄₁₆ fruit = 17 oz	0	2	?	152
	1 c diced	0	1	?	50
West Indian cherries *See* acerolas, *above*					

	Portion	Chol (mg)	Total Fat (g)	Satur'd Fat (g)	Total Calor
▪ **BRAND NAME**					
Birds Eye					
mixed fruit in syrup	5 oz	0	0	0	120
red raspberries in lite syrup	5 oz	0	1	?	100
strawberries, halved, in lite syrup	5 oz	0	0	0	90
strawberries, halved, in syrup	5 oz	0	0	0	120
Dromedary					
chopped dates	¼ c	?	0	?	130
pitted dates	5	?	0	?	100
Fresh Chef					
Tropical Delight fruit salad	7 oz	?	11	?	240
Mott's					
applesauce	4 oz	?	0	?	88
Mrs. Paul's					
apple fritters	2	?	13	?	270
Oregon Freeze Dry					
banana chips	¼ c	?	4	?	124
peaches	½ c	?	0	?	45
strawberries	½ c	?	0	?	60
Stouffer					
escalloped apples	4 oz	?	3	?	140

❑ **FRUIT & NUT SNACK MIXES** *See* SNACKS

❑ **FRUIT CHUTNEYS & RELISHES** *See* PICKLES, OLIVES, RELISHES, & CHUTNEYS

❑ **FRUIT SAUCES** *See* FRUIT, FRESH & PROCESSED

❑ **FRUIT SPREADS**

Fruit Butters

apple	1 T	0	tr	?	37
guava	1 T	?	0	0	39

	Portion	Chol (mg)	Total Fat (g)	Satur'd Fat (g)	Total Calor
Jams					
average, all varieties					
regular	1 T	0	tr	?	55
low-cal	1 T	0	tr	?	29
grape	1 T	0	tr	?	59
plum	1 T	0	tr	0	59
Jellies					
average, all varieties					
regular	1 T	0	tr	?	55
low-cal	1 T	0	0	0	27
blackberry	1 T	0	0	0	51
boysenberry	1 T	0	0	0	52
cherry	1 T	0	tr	?	52
currant	1 T	0	0	0	52
grape	1 T	0	tr	?	55
guava	1 T	0	tr	?	52
quince	1 T	0	tr	?	51
strawberry	1 T	0	0	?	51
Marmalades					
citrus	1 T	0	tr	?	51
orange	1 T	0	tr	?	56
papaya	1 T	0	0	0	57
Preserves					
apricot	1 T	0	tr	?	51
apricot-pineapple	1 T	0	tr	?	51
blackberry	1 T	0	tr	?	55
boysenberry	1 T	0	tr	?	54
peach	1 T	0	0	0	51

- **BRAND NAME**

Smucker's FRUIT BUTTERS					
apple	2 t	0	0	0	25
peach	2 t	0	0	0	30

JAMS, JELLIES, MARMALADES, & PRESERVES

all flavors					
regular	2 t	0	0	0	35
low-sugar or Slenderella	2 t	0	0	0	16
imitation grape jelly or strawberry jam, artificially sweetened	2 t	0	0	0	4

	Portion	Chol (mg)	Total Fat (g)	Satur'd Fat (g)	Total Calor

❑ GELATIN & GELATIN DESSERTS
See DESSERTS: CUSTARDS, GELATINS,
PUDDINGS, & PIE FILLINGS

❑ GRAINS *See* RICE & GRAINS,
PLAIN & PREPARED

❑ GRAVIES *See* SAUCES, GRAVIES,
& CONDIMENTS

❑ HAM *See* PORK, FRESH & CURED;
PROCESSED MEAT & POULTRY PRODUCTS

❑ HERBS & SPICES *See* SEASONINGS

❑ HONEY *See* SUGARS & SWEETENERS

❑ HOT DOGS *See* frankfurter, *under*
PROCESSED MEAT & POULTRY PRODUCTS

❑ ICE CREAM & ICE MILK
See DESSERTS, FROZEN

❑ INFANT & TODDLER FOODS

Baked Products

	Portion	Chol (mg)	Total Fat (g)	Satur'd Fat (g)	Total Calor
arrowroot cookies	1	tr	1	tr	24
	1 oz	tr	4	1	125
pretzels	1	?	tr	?	24
	1 oz	?	1	?	113
teething biscuits	1	?	1	?	43
	1 oz	?	1	?	111
zwieback	1	1	1	tr	30
	1 oz	6	3	1	121

	Portion	Chol (mg)	Total Fat (g)	Satur'd Fat (g)	Total Calor
Cereals, Hot & Cold					
barley					
dry	½ oz	?	tr	?	52
	1 T	?	tr	?	9
w/whole milk	1 oz	?	1	?	31
cereal & eggs, strained	about 4½ oz	66	2	1	112
	1 oz	15	tr	tr	25
cereal & egg yolks					
strained	about 4½ oz	81	2	1	66
	1 oz	18	1	tr	15
junior	about 7½ oz	?	4	1	110
	1 oz	?	1	tr	15
cereal, egg yolks, & bacon					
strained	about 4½ oz	?	7	?	101
	1 oz	?	1	?	22
junior	about 7½ oz	?	11	?	178
	1 oz	?	2	?	24
grits & egg yolks, strained	about 4½ oz	?	3	?	?
	1 oz	?	1	?	?
high protein					
dry	½ oz	?	1	?	51
	1 T	?	tr	?	9
w/whole milk	1 oz	?	1	?	31
high protein w/apple & orange					
dry	½ oz	?	1	?	53
	1 T	?	tr	?	9
w/whole milk	1 oz	?	1	?	32
mixed					
dry	½ oz	?	1	?	54
	1 T	?	tr	?	9
w/whole milk	1 oz	?	1	?	32
mixed w/applesauce & bananas					
strained	about 4.8 oz	?	1	?	111
	1 oz	?	tr	?	23
junior	about 7.8 oz	?	1	?	183
	1 oz	?	tr	?	24
mixed w/bananas					
dry	½ oz	?	1	?	56
	1 T	?	tr	?	9
w/whole milk	1 oz	?	1	?	33

	Portion	Chol (mg)	Total Fat (g)	Satur'd Fat (g)	Total Calor
mixed w/honey					
dry	½ oz	?	1	?	55
	1 T	?	tr	?	9
w/whole milk	1 oz	?	1	?	33
oatmeal					
dry	½ oz	?	1	?	56
	1 T	?	tr	?	10
w/whole milk	1 oz	?	1	?	33
oatmeal w/applesauce & bananas					
strained	about 4.8 oz	?	1	?	99
	1 oz	?	tr	?	21
junior	about 7.8 oz	?	2	?	165
	1 oz	?	tr	?	21
oatmeal w/bananas					
dry	½ oz	?	1	?	56
	1 T	?	tr	?	9
w/whole milk	1 oz	?	1	?	33
oatmeal w/honey					
dry	½ oz	?	1	?	55
	1 T	?	tr	?	9
w/whole milk	1 oz	?	1	?	33
rice					
dry	½ oz	?	1	?	56
	1 T	?	tr	?	9
w/whole milk	1 oz	?	1	?	33
rice w/applesauce & bananas, strained	about 4.8 oz	?	1	?	107
	1 oz	?	tr	?	23
rice w/bananas					
dry	½ oz	?	1	?	57
	1 T	?	tr	?	10
w/whole milk	1 oz	?	1	?	33
rice w/honey					
dry	½ oz	?	tr	?	56
	1 T	?	tr	?	9
w/whole milk	1 oz	?	1	?	33
rice w/mixed fruit, junior	about 7.8 oz	?	1	?	186
	1 oz	?	tr	?	24

Desserts

	Portion	Chol (mg)	Total Fat (g)	Satur'd Fat (g)	Total Calor
apple Betty					
strained	about 4.8 oz	?	0	?	97
	1 oz	?	0	?	20
junior	about 7.8 oz	?	0	?	153
	1 oz	?	0	?	20

	Portion	Chol (mg)	Total Fat (g)	Satur'd Fat (g)	Total Calor
caramel pudding					
strained	about 4.8 oz	?	1	?	104
	1 oz	?	tr	?	22
junior	about 7½ oz	?	2	?	167
	1 oz	?	tr	?	22
cherry vanilla pudding					
strained	about 4.8 oz	?	tr	?	91
	1 oz	?	tr	?	19
junior	about 7.8 oz	?	tr	?	152
	1 oz	?	tr	?	20
chocolate custard pudding					
strained	about 4½ oz	?	2	?	107
	1 oz	?	1	?	24
junior	about 7.8 oz	?	4	?	195
	1 oz	?	1	?	25
cottage cheese w/pine-apple					
strained	about 4.8 oz	?	1	?	94
	1 oz	?	tr	?	20
junior	about 7.8 oz	?	2	?	172
	1 oz	?	tr	?	22
Dutch apple					
strained	about 4.8 oz	?	1	1	92
	1 oz	?	tr	tr	19
junior	about 7.8 oz	?	2	1	151
	1 oz	?	tr	tr	19
fruit dessert					
strained	about 4.8 oz	?	0	?	79
	1 oz	?	0	?	17
junior	about 7.8 oz	?	0	?	138
	1 oz	?	0	?	18
orange pudding, strained	about 4.8 oz	?	1	?	108
	1 oz	?	tr	?	23
peach cobbler					
strained	about 4.8 oz	?	0	?	88
	1 oz	?	0	?	18

	Portion	Chol (mg)	Total Fat (g)	Satur'd Fat (g)	Total Calor
peach cobbler *(cont.)*					
junior	about 7.8 oz	?	0	?	147
	1 oz	?	0	?	19
peach melba					
strained	about 4.8 oz	?	0	?	81
	1 oz	?	0	?	17
junior	about 7.8 oz	?	0	?	132
	1 oz	?	0	?	17
pineapple orange, strained	about 4½ oz	?	0	?	89
	1 oz	?	0	?	20
pineapple pudding					
strained	about 4½ oz	?	tr	?	104
	1 oz	?	tr	?	23
junior	about 7.8 oz	?	1	?	192
	1 oz	?	tr	?	25
tropical fruit, junior	about 7.8 oz	?	0	?	131
	1 oz	?	0	?	17
vanilla custard pudding					
strained	about 4½ oz	?	3	1	109
	1 oz	?	1	tr	24
junior	about 7.8 oz	?	5	3	196
	1 oz	?	1	tr	25

Dinners, Regular

	Portion	Chol (mg)	Total Fat (g)	Satur'd Fat (g)	Total Calor
beef & egg noodles					
strained	about 4½ oz	?	2	?	68
	1 oz	?	1	?	15
junior	about 7½ oz	?	4	?	122
	1 oz	?	1	?	16
beef & rice, toddler	about 6.2 oz	?	5	?	146
	1 oz	?	1	?	23
beef lasagna, toddler	about 6.2 oz	?	4	?	137
	1 oz	?	1	?	22
beef stew, toddler	about 6.2 oz	22	2	1	90
	1 oz	4	tr	tr	14

	Portion	Chol (mg)	Total Fat (g)	Satur'd Fat (g)	Total Calor
chicken & noodles					
strained	about 4½ oz	?	2	?	67
	1 oz	?	tr	?	15
junior	about 7½ oz	?	3	?	109
	1 oz	?	tr	?	15
chicken soup, strained	about 4½ oz	?	2	?	64
	1 oz	?	1	?	14
chicken soup, cream of, strained	about 4½ oz	?	2	?	74
	1 oz	?	1	?	16
chicken stew, toddler	about 6 oz	49	6	2	132
	1 oz	8	1	tr	22
lamb & noodles, junior	about 1½ oz	?	5	?	138
	1 oz	?	1	?	18
macaroni & bacon, toddler	about 7½ oz	?	7	?	160
	1 oz	?	1	?	21
macaroni & cheese					
strained	about 4½ oz	?	3	?	76
	1 oz	?	1	?	17
junior	about 7½ oz	?	4	?	130
	1 oz	?	1	?	17
macaroni & ham, junior	about 7½ oz	?	3	?	127
	1 oz	?	tr	?	17
macaroni, tomato, & beef					
strained	about 4½ oz	?	1	?	71
	1 oz	?	tr	?	16
junior	about 7½ oz	?	2	?	125
	1 oz	?	tr	?	17
mixed vegetables					
strained	about 4½ oz	?	tr	?	52
	1 oz	?	0	?	11
junior	about 7½ oz	?	tr	?	71
	1 oz	?	0	?	9
spaghetti, tomato, & meat					
junior	about 7½ oz	?	3	?	135
	1 oz	?	tr	?	18
toddler	about 6.2 oz	?	2	?	133
	1 oz	?	tr	?	21

	Portion	Chol (mg)	Total Fat (g)	Satur'd Fat (g)	Total Calor
split peas & ham, junior	about 7½ oz	?	3	?	152
	1 oz	?	tr	?	20
turkey & rice					
strained	about 4½ oz	13	2	1	63
	1 oz	3	tr	tr	14
junior	about 7½ oz	?	3	1	104
	1 oz	?	tr	tr	14
vegetables & bacon					
strained	about 4½ oz	4	4	2	88
	1 oz	1	1	tr	19
junior	about 7½ oz	?	8	3	150
	1 oz	?	1	tr	20
vegetables & beef					
strained	about 4½ oz	?	3	?	67
	1 oz	?	1	?	15
junior	about 7½ oz	?	4	?	113
	1 oz	?	1	?	15
vegetables & chicken					
strained	about 4½ oz	?	1	?	55
	1 oz	?	tr	?	12
junior	about 7½ oz	?	2	?	106
	1 oz	?	tr	?	14
vegetables & ham					
strained	about 4½ oz	?	2	?	62
	1 oz	?	1	?	14
junior	about 7½ oz	?	4	?	110
	1 oz	?	1	?	15
toddler	about 6.2 oz	14	5	2	128
	1 oz	2	1	tr	21
vegetables & lamb					
strained	about 4½ oz	?	3	?	67
	1 oz	?	1	?	15
junior	about 7½ oz	?	4	?	108
	1 oz	?	1	?	14
vegetables & liver					
strained	about 4½ oz	?	1	?	50
	1 oz	?	tr	?	11

	Portion	Chol (mg)	Total Fat (g)	Satur'd Fat (g)	Total Calor.
junior	about 7½ oz	?	1	?	93
	1 oz	?	tr	?	12
vegetables & turkey					
strained	about 4½ oz	?	2	?	54
	1 oz	?	tr	?	12
junior	about 7½ oz	?	3	?	101
	1 oz	?	tr	?	13
toddler	about 6.2 oz	?	6	?	141
	1 oz	?	1	?	23
vegetables, dumplings, & beef					
strained	about 4½ oz	?	1	?	61
	1 oz	?	tr	?	14
junior	about 7½ oz	?	2	?	103
	1 oz	?	tr	?	14
vegetables, noodles, & chicken					
strained	about 4½ oz	?	3	?	81
	1 oz	?	1	?	18
junior	about 7½ oz	?	5	?	137
	1 oz	?	1	?	18
vegetables, noodles, & turkey					
strained	about 4½ oz	?	2	?	56
	1 oz	?	tr	?	12
junior	about 7½ oz	?	3	?	110
	1 oz	?	tr	?	15

Dinners, High in Meat or Cheese

	Portion	Chol (mg)	Total Fat (g)	Satur'd Fat (g)	Total Calor.
beef w/vegetables					
strained	about 4½ oz	?	5	?	96
	1 oz	?	1	?	21
junior	about 4½ oz	?	6	?	108
	1 oz	?	1	?	24

	Portion	Chol (mg)	Total Fat (g)	Satur'd Fat (g)	Total Calor
chicken w/vegetables					
strained	about 4½ oz	?	5	?	100
	1 oz	?	1	?	22
junior	about 4½ oz	?	7	?	117
	1 oz	?	2	?	26
cottage cheese w/pine-apple, strained	about 4.8 oz	?	3	?	157
	1 oz	?	1	?	33
ham w/vegetables					
strained	about 4½ oz	?	4	2	97
	1 oz	?	1	tr	21
junior	about 4½ oz	23	4	1	98
	1 oz	5	1	tr	22
turkey w/vegetables					
strained	about 4½ oz	?	6	?	111
	1 oz	?	1	?	25
junior	about 4½ oz	?	6	?	115
	1 oz	?	1	?	25
veal w/vegetables					
strained	about 4½ oz	?	3	?	89
	1 oz	?	1	?	20
junior	about 4½ oz	?	4	?	93
	1 oz	?	1	?	21

Fruit
See also Desserts, above

all types	varies	?	0 or tr	?	varies

Fruit Juices

all types	varies	?	0 or tr	?	varies

Meats & Egg Yolks

beef					
strained	about 3½ oz	?	5	3	106
	1 oz	?	2	1	30
junior	about 3½ oz	?	5	3	105
	1 oz	?	1	1	30
beef w/beef heart, strained	about 3½ oz	?	4	2	93
	1 oz	?	1	1	27

	Portion	Chol. (mg)	Total Fat (g)	Satur'd Fat (g)	Total Calor
chicken					
strained	about 3½ oz	?	8	2	128
	1 oz	?	2	1	37
junior	about 3½ oz	?	10	2	148
	1 oz	?	3	1	42
chicken sticks, junior	2½ oz	?	10	?	134
	1 stick = 0.35 oz	?	1	?	19
egg yolks, strained	about 3.3 oz	739	16	5	191
	1 oz	223	5	1	58
ham					
strained	about 3½ oz	?	6	2	110
	1 oz	?	2	1	32
junior	about 3½ oz	?	7	2	123
	1 oz	?	2	1	35
lamb					
strained	about 3½ oz	?	5	2	102
	1 oz	?	1	1	29
junior	about 3½ oz	?	5	3	111
	1 oz	?	2	1	32
liver, strained	about 3½ oz	182	4	1	100
	1 oz	52	1	tr	29
meat sticks, junior	2½ oz	?	10	4	130
	1 stick = 0.35 oz	?	2	1	18
pork, strained	about 3½ oz	?	7	2	123
	1 oz	?	2	1	35
turkey					
strained	about 3½ oz	?	6	2	113
	1 oz	?	2	1	32
junior	about 3½ oz	?	7	2	128
	1 oz	?	2	1	37
turkey sticks, junior	2½ oz	?	10	?	129
	1 stick = 0.35 oz	?	1	?	18
veal					
strained	about 3½ oz	?	5	2	100
	1 oz	?	1	1	29
junior	about 3½ oz	?	5	2	109
	1 oz	?	1	1	31

	Portion	Chol (mg)	Total Fat (g)	Satur'd Fat (g)	Total Calor
Vegetables					
beans, green					
plain					
strained	about 4½ oz	?	tr	?	32
	1 oz	?	0	?	7
junior	about 7.3 oz	?	tr	?	51
	1 oz	?	0	?	7
buttered					
strained	about 4½ oz	?	1	?	42
	1 oz	?	tr	?	9
junior	about 7.3 oz	?	2	?	67
	1 oz	?	tr	?	9
creamed, junior	about 7½ oz	?	1	?	68
	1 oz	?	tr	?	9
beets, strained	about 4½ oz	?	tr	?	43
	1 oz	?	0	?	10
carrots					
plain					
strained	about 4½ oz	?	tr	?	34
	1 oz	?	0	?	8
junior	about 7½ oz	?	tr	?	67
	1 oz	?	0	?	9
buttered					
strained	about 4½ oz	?	1	?	46
	1 oz	?	tr	?	10
junior	about 7½ oz	?	1	?	70
	1 oz	?	tr	?	9
corn, creamed					
strained	about 4½ oz	?	1	?	73
	1 oz	?	tr	?	16
junior	about 7½ oz	?	1	?	138
	1 oz	?	tr	?	18
garden vegetables, strained	about 4½ oz	?	tr	?	48
	1 oz	?	tr	?	11

	Portion	Chol (mg)	Total Fat (g)	Satur'd Fat (g)	Total Calor
mixed vegetables					
strained	about 4½ oz	?	1	?	52
	1 oz	?	tr	?	11
junior	about 7½ oz	?	1	?	88
	1 oz	?	tr	?	12
peas					
plain, strained	about 4½ oz	?	tr	?	52
	1 oz	?	tr	?	11
buttered					
strained	about 4½ oz	?	1	?	72
	1 oz	?	tr	?	16
junior	about 7.3 oz	?	3	?	123
	1 oz	?	tr	?	17
creamed, strained	about 4½ oz	?	2	?	68
	1 oz	?	1	?	15
spinach, creamed					
strained	about 4½ oz	?	2	?	48
	1 oz	?	tr	?	11
junior	about 7½ oz	?	3	?	90
	1 oz	?	tr	?	12
squash					
plain					
strained	about 4½ oz	?	tr	?	30
	1 oz	?	tr	?	7
junior	about 7½ oz	?	tr	?	51
	1 oz	?	tr	?	7
buttered					
strained	about 4½ oz	?	tr	?	37
	1 oz	?	tr	?	8
junior	about 7½ oz	?	1	?	63
	1 oz	?	tr	?	8
sweet potatoes					
plain					
strained	about 4.8 oz	?	tr	?	77
	1 oz	?	0	?	16
junior	about 7.8 oz	?	tr	?	133
	1 oz	?	0	?	17

	Portion	Chol (mg)	Total Fat (g)	Satur'd Fat (g)	Total Calor
sweet potatoes *(cont.)*					
buttered					
strained	about 4.8 oz	?	1	?	76
	1 oz	?	tr	?	16
junior	about 7.8 oz	?	2	?	126
	1 oz	?	tr	?	16

▪ BRAND NAME

Beech-Nut
STAGE 1

Cereal

barley	½ oz dry	?	0	?	50
	½ oz dry + 2.4 fl oz milk	?	3	?	100
oatmeal	½ oz dry	?	1	?	50
	½ oz dry + 2.4 fl oz milk	?	4	?	100
rice	½ oz dry	?	1	?	60
	½ oz dry + 2.4 fl oz milk	?	3	?	100

Fruit & Fruit Dishes

bartlett pears	4½ oz	?	0	?	70
Chiquita bananas	4½ oz	?	0	?	100
golden delicious apple-sauce	4½ oz	?	0	?	60
yellow cling peaches	4½ oz	?	0	?	60

Fruit Juices

apple	4.2 fl oz	?	0	?	60
pear	4.2 fl oz	?	0	?	60
white grape	4.2 fl oz	?	0	?	80

Meat

beef	3½ oz	?	8	?	120
chicken	3½ oz	?	6	?	110
lamb	3½ oz	?	8	?	130
turkey	3½ oz	?	7	?	120
veal	3½ oz	?	7	?	120

Vegetables

butternut squash	4½ oz	?	0	?	40
green beans	4½ oz	?	0	?	40
regal imperial carrots	4½ oz	?	0	?	40
sweet potatoes	4½ oz	?	0	?	70

	Portion	Chol (mg)	Total Fat (g)	Satur'd Fat (g)	Total Calor
tender sweet peas	4½ oz	?	0	?	70

STAGE 2

Cereals

	Portion	Chol (mg)	Total Fat (g)	Satur'd Fat (g)	Total Calor
Hi-Protein	½ oz dry	?	1	?	50
	½ oz dry + 2.4 fl oz milk	?	3	?	90
mixed	½ oz dry	?	1	?	50
	½ oz dry + 2.4 fl oz milk	?	3	?	100
w/applesauce & bananas	4½ oz	?	0	?	80
oatmeal					
w/applesauce & bananas	4½ oz	?	1	?	90
w/bananas	½ oz dry	?	1	?	60
	½ oz dry + 2.4 fl oz milk	?	3	?	100
rice					
w/applesauce & bananas	4½ oz	?	0	?	100
w/bananas	½ oz dry	?	0	?	60
	½ oz dry + 2.4 fl oz milk	?	3	?	100

Desserts

	Portion	Chol (mg)	Total Fat (g)	Satur'd Fat (g)	Total Calor
banana custard	4½ oz	?	1	?	120
banana pineapple	4½ oz	?	0	?	100
Dutch apple	4½ oz	?	0	?	80
guava tropical fruit	4½ oz	?	0	?	100
mango tropical fruit	4½ oz	?	0	?	90
papaya tropical fruit	4½ oz	?	0	?	80
vanilla custard	4½ oz	?	3	?	130

Fruit & Dairy

	Portion	Chol (mg)	Total Fat (g)	Satur'd Fat (g)	Total Calor
cottage cheese w/pine-apple	4½ oz	?	1	?	110
mixed fruit & yogurt	4½ oz	?	1	?	110
peaches & yogurt	4½ oz	?	1	?	110

Fruit & Fruit Dishes

	Portion	Chol (mg)	Total Fat (g)	Satur'd Fat (g)	Total Calor
apples & grapes	4½ oz	?	0	?	90
apples & strawberries	4½ oz	?	0	?	90
applesauce & apricots	4½ oz	?	0	?	60
applesauce & bananas	4½ oz	?	0	?	60
applesauce & cherries	4½ oz	?	0	?	70
apples, mandarin oranges, & bananas	4½ oz	?	0	?	90

	Portion	Chol (mg)	Total Fat (g)	Satur'd Fat (g)	Total Calor
apples, peaches, & strawberries	4½ oz	?	0	?	100
apples, pears, & bananas	4½ oz	?	0	?	90
apricots w/pears & applesauce	4½ oz	?	0	?	70
bananas w/pears & applesauce	4½ oz	?	0	?	90
bartlett pears & pineapple	4½ oz	?	0	?	70
Fruit Dessert	4½ oz	?	0	?	80
Island Fruits	4½ oz	?	0	?	90
pears & applesauce	4½ oz	?	0	?	70
plums w/rice	4½ oz	?	0	?	110
prunes w/pears	4½ oz	?	0	?	120

Juice

Juice Plus	4 fl oz	?	0	?	80

Main Courses

beef & egg noodles w/vegetables	4½ oz	?	4	?	90
Beef Dinner Supreme	4½ oz	?	7	?	120
chicken & rice w/vegetables	4½ oz	?	3	?	80
chicken noodle w/vegetables	4½ oz	?	3	?	90
macaroni, tomato, & beef	4½ oz	?	3	?	90
Turkey Dinner Supreme	4½ oz	?	5	?	110
turkey rice w/vegetables	4½ oz	?	2	?	70
vegetable beef	4½ oz	?	3	?	90
vegetable chicken	4½ oz	?	3	?	90
vegetable ham	4½ oz	?	3	?	90
vegetable lamb	4½ oz	?	3	?	90

Vegetables

creamed corn	4½ oz	?	0	?	90
garden vegetables	4½ oz	?	0	?	60
mixed vegetables	4½ oz	?	0	?	50
peas & carrots	4½ oz	?	0	?	60

STAGE 3

Custard

banana	7½ oz	?	2	?	200
vanilla	7½ oz	?	5	?	210

Fruit & Dairy

cottage cheese w/pineapple	7½ oz	?	2	?	190
mixed fruit & yogurt	7½ oz	?	1	?	170

	Portion	Chol (mg)	Total Fat (g)	Satur'd Fat (g)	Total Calor
peaches & yogurt	7½ oz	?	2	?	190

FRUIT & FRUIT DISHES

apples & grapes	7½ oz	?	0	?	190
apples & strawberries	7½ oz	?	0	?	160
applesauce	7½ oz	?	0	?	100
applesauce & bananas	7½ oz	?	0	?	110
applesauce & cherries	7½ oz	?	0	?	110
apples, mandarin oranges, & bananas	7½ oz	?	0	?	150
apples, peaches, & strawberries	7½ oz	?	0	?	160
apples, pears, & bananas	7½ oz	?	0	?	160
apricots w/pears & apples	7½ oz	?	0	?	120
bananas w/pears & apples	7½ oz	?	0	?	160
bartlett pears	7½ oz	?	0	?	110
bartlett pears & pineapple	7½ oz	?	0	?	120
Fruit Dessert	7½ oz	?	0	?	130
Island Fruits	7½ oz	?	0	?	150
peaches	7½ oz	?	0	?	150

Main Courses & Dinners

beef & egg noodles w/vegetables	7½ oz	?	5	?	150
Beef Dinner Supreme	7½ oz	?	9	?	180
chicken noodles w/vegetables	7½ oz	?	4	?	140
macaroni, tomato, & beef	7½ oz	?	5	?	150
spaghetti, tomato, & beef	7½ oz	?	5	?	170
Turkey Dinner Supreme	7½ oz	?	8	?	190
turkey rice w/vegetables	7½ oz	?	4	?	130
vegetable bacon	7½ oz	?	9	?	180
vegetable beef	7½ oz	?	5	?	150
vegetable chicken	7½ oz	?	5	?	140
vegetable lamb	7½ oz	?	5	?	140

Vegetables

carrots	7½ oz	?	0	?	60
green beans	7½ oz	?	0	?	60
mixed vegetables	7½ oz	?	0	?	90
sweet potatoes	7½ oz	?	0	?	120

UNSTAGED

Juices

apple	4 fl oz	?	0	?	60
apple banana	4.2 fl oz	?	0	?	60
apple cherry	4.2 fl oz	?	0	?	50
apple cranberry	4.2 fl oz	?	0	?	60
apple grape	4.2 fl oz	?	0	?	60
apple pear	4.2 fl oz	?	0	?	60

	Portion	Chol (mg)	Total Fat (g)	Satur'd Fat (g)	Total Calor
mixed fruit	4.2 fl oz	?	0	?	60
orange	4.2 fl oz	?	0	?	60
pear	4 fl oz	?	0	?	60
tropical blend	4 fl oz	?	0	?	70

TABLE TIME

Main Courses

beef stew	6 oz	?	4	?	140
pasta squares in meat sauce	6 oz	?	4	?	140
spaghetti rings in meat sauce	6 oz	?	4	?	160
vegetable stew w/chicken	6 oz	?	8	?	190

Soups

Hearty chicken w/stars	6 oz	?	9	?	180
Hearty vegetable	6 oz	?	0	?	70

Gerber
BAKED GOODS

animal crackers	4	?	2	?	50
animal-shaped cookies	2	tr	2	?	60
arrowroot cookies	2	tr	2	?	50
pretzels	2	0	0	?	50
Toddler Biter biscuits	1	tr	1	?	50
vanilla number cookies	4	?	3	?	60
zwieback toast	2	tr	2	?	60

CHUNKY PRODUCTS

beef & egg noodles w/vegetables	6 oz	13	4	?	130
Homestyle noodles & beef	6 oz	?	6	?	150
macaroni alphabets w/beef & tomato sauce	6¼ oz	7	3	?	130
noodles & chicken w/carrots & peas	6 oz	20	2	?	100
potatoes & ham	6 oz	7	4	?	110
rice w/beef & tomato sauce	6¼ oz	?	5	?	150
saucy rice w/chicken	6 oz	?	2	?	110
spaghetti tomato sauce & beef	6¼ oz	10	5	?	160
vegetables & beef	6¼ oz	10	5	?	140
vegetables & chicken	6¼ oz	16	5	?	140
vegetables & ham	6¼ oz	10	4	?	120
vegetables & turkey	6¼ oz	20	3	?	110

	Portion	Chol (mg)	Total Fat (g)	Satur'd Fat (g)	Total Calor
DRY CEREALS, READY-TO-SERVE					
barley	½ oz dry	?	1	?	60
	½ oz dry + 2.4 fl oz milk	?	4	?	110
high protein	½ oz dry	?	1	?	50
	½ oz dry + 2.4 fl oz milk	?	4	?	100
w/apple & orange	½ oz dry	?	1	?	60
	½ oz dry + 2.4 fl oz milk	?	4	?	100
mixed	½ oz dry	?	1	?	50
	½ oz dry + 2.4 fl oz milk	?	4	?	100
w/banana	½ oz dry	?	1	?	60
	½ oz dry + 2.4 fl oz milk	?	4	?	100
oatmeal	½ oz dry	?	1	?	50
	½ oz dry + 2.4 fl oz milk	?	4	?	100
w/banana	½ oz dry	?	1	?	60
	½ oz dry + 2.4 fl oz milk	?	4	?	100
rice	½ oz dry	?	1	?	60
	½ oz dry + 2.4 fl oz milk	?	4	?	100
w/banana	½ oz dry	?	1	?	60
	½ oz dry + 2.4 fl oz milk	?	4	?	100
STRAINED FOODS					
Cereals w/Fruit					
mixed w/applesauce & bananas	4½ oz	?	1	?	100
oatmeal w/applesauce & bananas	4½ oz	?	1	?	100
rice w/applesauce & bananas	4½ oz	?	1	?	100

	Portion	Chol (mg)	Total Fat (g)	Satur'd Fat (g)	Total Calor
Desserts					
banana apple	4½ oz	0	1	?	90
cherry vanilla pudding	4½ oz	3	1	?	90
chocolate custard pudding	4½ oz	14	2	?	110
Dutch apple	4½ oz	4	2	?	100
fruit	4½ oz	0	1	?	100
Hawaiian Delight	4½ oz	2	1	?	120
orange pudding	4½ oz	11	1	?	110
peach cobbler	4½ oz	0	1	?	100
vanilla custard pudding	4½ oz	15	1	?	100
Dinners, Regular					
beef egg noodle	4½ oz	6	3	?	90
cereal egg yolk bacon	4½ oz	64	5	?	100
chicken noodle	4½ oz	10	2	?	80
cream of chicken soup	4½ oz	12	2	?	70
macaroni cheese	4½ oz	3	3	?	90
macaroni tomato beef	4½ oz	3	2	?	80
turkey rice	4½ oz	15	3	?	80
vegetable bacon	4½ oz	4	5	?	100
vegetable beef	4½ oz	5	3	?	80
vegetable chicken	4½ oz	7	2	?	80
vegetable ham	4½ oz	4	3	?	80
vegetable lamb	4½ oz	3	4	?	90
vegetable liver	4½ oz	29	1	?	60
vegetable turkey	4½ oz	12	2	?	70
Dinners, High in Meat					
beef w/vegetables	4½ oz	14	6	?	120
chicken w/vegetables	4½ oz	21	8	?	140
ham w/vegetables	4½ oz	12	4	?	100
turkey w/vegetables	4½ oz	19	7	?	130
veal w/vegetables	4½ oz	12	4	?	100
Fruit & Tropical Fruit					
apple blueberry	4½ oz	?	1	?	60
applesauce	4½ oz	?	0	?	60
applesauce apricot	4½ oz	?	1	?	70
applesauce w/pineapple	4½ oz	?	1	?	60
apricots w/tapioca	4½ oz	?	1	?	90
bananas w/pineapple & tapioca	4½ oz	?	1	?	70
bananas w/tapioca	4½ oz	?	0	?	100
guava w/tapioca	4½ oz	?	1	?	90
mango w/tapioca	4½ oz	?	1	?	90
papaya w/tapioca	4½ oz	?	1	?	80
peaches	4½ oz	?	1	?	90
pear pineapple	4½ oz	?	1	?	80

	Portion	Chol (mg)	Total Fat (g)	Satur'd Fat (g)	Total Calor
pears	4½ oz	?	1	?	80
plums w/tapioca	4½ oz	?	1	?	100
prunes w/tapioca	4½ oz	?	1	?	100
Tropical Fruit Medley	4½ oz	?	1	?	80

Juices

apple	4.2 oz	?	0	?	60
apple apricot	4.2 oz	?	0	?	60
apple banana	4.2 oz	?	1	?	70
apple cherry	4.2 oz	?	0	?	60
apple grape	4.2 oz	?	0	?	60
apple peach	4.2 oz	?	0	?	60
apple pineapple	4.2 oz	?	0	?	60
apple plum	4.2 oz	?	0	?	60
apple prune	4.2 oz	?	0	?	70
mixed fruit	4.2 oz	?	1	?	70
orange	4.2 oz	?	1	?	70
orange apple	4.2 oz	?	1	?	70
pear	4.2 oz	?	0	?	60

Meats & Egg Yolks

beef	3½ oz	29	5	?	100
beef liver	3½ oz	121	4	?	100
chicken	3½ oz	61	9	?	140
egg yolks	3½ oz	585	17	?	190
ham	3½ oz	24	6	?	110
lamb	3½ oz	38	5	?	100
pork	3½ oz	35	6	?	110
turkey	3½ oz	59	8	?	130
veal	3½ oz	26	5	?	100

Vegetables

beets	4½ oz	?	0	?	50
carrots	4½ oz	?	1	?	40
creamed corn	4½ oz	?	1	?	80
creamed spinach	4½ oz	?	1	?	60
garden vegetables	4½ oz	?	1	?	50
green beans	4½ oz	?	1	?	50
mixed vegetables	4½ oz	?	1	?	50
peas	4½ oz	?	1	?	60
squash	4½ oz	?	1	?	40
sweet potatoes	4½ oz	?	1	?	80

FIRST FOODS

Fruit

applesauce	2½ oz	?	0	?	30
bananas	2½ oz	?	0	?	60
peaches	2½ oz	?	0	?	30
pears	2½ oz	?	0	?	40

	Portion	Chol (mg)	Total Fat (g)	Satur'd Fat (g)	Total Calor
Vegetables					
carrots	2½ oz	?	1	?	30
green beans	2½ oz	?	0	?	20
peas	2½ oz	?	1	?	40
squash	2½ oz	?	0	?	20
sweet potatoes	2½ oz	?	0	?	50
JUNIOR FOODS					
Cereals w/Fruit					
mixed w/applesauce & bananas	7½ oz	?	2	?	170
oatmeal w/applesauce & bananas	7½ oz	?	2	?	160
rice w/mixed fruit	7½ oz	?	1	?	170
Desserts					
banana apple	7½ oz	0	1	?	150
cherry vanilla pudding	7½ oz	7	1	?	150
Dutch apple	7½ oz	9	2	?	160
fruit	7½ oz	0	1	?	160
Hawaiian Delight	7½ oz	3	1	?	190
peach cobbler	7½ oz	0	1	?	160
vanilla custard pudding	7½ oz	29	2	?	190
Dinners, Regular					
beef egg noodle	7½ oz	12	4	?	140
chicken noodle	7½ oz	18	3	?	120
macaroni tomato beef	7½ oz	8	3	?	130
spaghetti tomato sauce beef	7½ oz	9	2	?	140
split peas ham	7½ oz	5	3	?	150
turkey rice	7½ oz	24	4	?	120
vegetable bacon	7½ oz	7	8	?	180
vegetable beef	7½ oz	9	4	?	140
vegetable chicken	7½ oz	17	3	?	120
vegetable ham	7½ oz	9	4	?	140
vegetable lamb	7½ oz	6	5	?	140
vegetable turkey	7½ oz	24	3	?	120
Dinners, High in Meat					
beef w/vegetables	4½ oz	15	7	?	130
chicken w/vegetables	4½ oz	26	7	?	130
ham w/vegetables	4½ oz	14	4	?	110
turkey w/vegetables	4½ oz	20	8	?	140
veal w/vegetables	4½ oz	12	4	?	110

	Portion	Chol (mg)	Total Fat (g)	Satur'd Fat (g)	Total Calor
Fruit					
apple blueberry	7½ oz	?	1	?	110
applesauce	7½ oz	?	1	?	100
applesauce apricot	7½ oz	?	1	?	110
apricots w/tapioca	7½ oz	?	1	?	160
bananas w/pineapple & tapioca	7½ oz	?	1	?	110
bananas w/tapioca	7½ oz	?	0	?	160
peaches	7½ oz	?	1	?	140
pear pineapple	7½ oz	?	1	?	120
pears	7½ oz	?	1	?	120
plums w/tapioca	7½ oz	?	1	?	160
Meats					
beef	3½ oz	27	5	?	110
chicken	3½ oz	58	9	?	140
ham	3½ oz	29	7	?	120
lamb	3½ oz	40	5	?	100
turkey	3½ oz	53	8	?	130
veal	3½ oz	27	5	?	100
Vegetables					
carrots	7½ oz	?	1	?	60
creamed corn	7½ oz	?	1	?	130
creamed green beans	7½ oz	?	1	?	100
mixed vegetables	7½ oz	?	1	?	90
peas	7½ oz	?	1	?	110
squash	7½ oz	?	1	?	70
sweet potatoes	7½ oz	?	1	?	140
TODDLER FOODS					
Cereals					
Toasted Oat Rings	½ oz dry	?	1	?	60
	½ oz dry + 2.7 fl oz milk	?	4	?	110
Juices					
all	4 oz	?	0	0	60
Meat & Poultry Sticks					
chicken	2½ oz	65	8	?	120
meat	2½ oz	33	7	?	110
turkey	2½ oz	61	9	?	120
Health Valley					
instant brown rice cereal	½ oz or 2 T	0	1	?	60

	Portion	Chol (mg)	Total Fat (g)	Satur'd Fat (g)	Total Calor
sprouted cereal w/bananas	½ oz or 2 T	0	1	?	50
Nabisco					
zwieback teething toast	2	?	1	?	60

❑ **JAMS & JELLIES** *See* FRUIT SPREADS

❑ **JUICE, FROZEN** *See* DESSERTS, FROZEN

❑ **JUICES & JUICE DRINKS**
See BEVERAGES

❑ **LAMB, VEAL,
& MISCELLANEOUS MEATS**

Lamb, Cooked

	Portion	Chol (mg)	Total Fat (g)	Satur'd Fat (g)	Total Calor
lamb chops (3/lb w/bone)					
lean & fat					
arm, braised	2.2 oz	77	15	7	220
loin, broiled	2.8 oz	78	16	7	235
rib	3½ oz	70	37	?	423
lean only					
arm, braised	1.7 oz	59	7	3	135
loin, broiled	2.3 oz	60	6	3	140
leg of lamb, roasted					
lean & fat	3 oz	78	13	6	205
lean only	2.6 oz	65	6	2	140
rib, roasted					
lean & fat	3 oz	77	26	12	315
lean only	2 oz	50	7	3	130

Veal, Cooked

	Portion	Chol (mg)	Total Fat (g)	Satur'd Fat (g)	Total Calor
arm steak, lean & fat	3½ oz	90	19	?	298
blade, lean & fat	3½ oz	90	17	?	276
breast, stewed w/gravy	2.6 oz	?	19	?	256
cutlet, medium fat, bone removed					
braised or broiled	3 oz	109	9	4	185
breaded	3½ oz	?	15	?	319
flank, medium fat, stewed	3½ oz	90	32	?	390
foreshank, medium fat, stewed	3½ oz	90	10	?	216

	Portion	Chol (mg)	Total Fat (g)	Satur'd Fat (g)	Total Calor
loin chop, lean & fat	3½ oz	90	36	?	421
plate, medium fat, stewed	3½ oz	90	21	?	303
rib, roasted	3 oz	109	14	6	230

Other Meats

	Portion	Chol (mg)	Total Fat (g)	Satur'd Fat (g)	Total Calor
alligator, raw	3½ oz	?	4	?	232
armadillo, raw	3½ oz	?	5	?	172
frog legs					
raw	4 large	50	tr	?	73
flour-coated & fried	6 large	?	29	?	418
goat, raw	3½ oz	?	9	?	165
guinea pig, raw	3½ oz	?	2	?	96
hare, raw	3½ oz	?	5	?	135
opossum, roasted	3½ oz	?	10	?	221
rabbit, stewed	3½ oz	?	10	?	216
reindeer, forequarter, raw	3½ oz	?	9	?	178
snail, raw	3½ oz	?	1	?	90
turtle, green, raw	3½ oz	?	1	?	89
venison, roasted	3½ oz	?	2	?	146
whale meat, raw	3½ oz	15	8	?	156

❑ LEGUMES & LEGUME PRODUCTS

Beans

	Portion	Chol (mg)	Total Fat (g)	Satur'd Fat (g)	Total Calor
adzuki					
boiled	½ c	0	tr	?	147
canned, sweetened	½ c	0	tr	?	351
yokan (sugar & bean confection)	1½ oz	0	tr	tr	36
black, boiled	½ c	0	tr	tr	113
black turtle soup					
boiled	1 c	0	1	tr	241
canned	½ c	0	tr	tr	109
broad					
raw	½ c	0	1	tr	256
boiled	½ c	0	tr	tr	93
canned, solids & liquids	½ c	0	tr	tr	91
cannellini See kidney, *below*					
cranberry					
boiled	½ c	0	tr	tr	120
canned, solids & liquids	½ c	0	tr	tr	108
fava See broad, *above*					
French, boiled	½ c	0	1	tr	111
garbanzo See chickpeas, *under* Peas & Lentils, *below*					
great northern					
boiled	½ c	0	tr	tr	104
canned, solids & liquids	½ c	0	1	tr	150

	Portion	Chol (mg)	Total Fat (g)	Satur'd Fat (g)	Total Calor
green gram *See* mung, *below*					
hyacinth, boiled	½ c	0	1	?	114
kidney					
all types					
boiled	½ c	0	tr	tr	112
canned, solids & liquids	½ c	0	tr	tr	104
California red, boiled	½ c	0	tr	tr	109
red					
boiled	½ c	0	tr	tr	112
canned, solids & liquids	½ c	0	tr	tr	108
royal red, boiled	½ c	0	tr	tr	108
lima					
baby					
boiled	½ c	0	tr	tr	115
frozen, boiled, drained	10 oz pkg	0	1	tr	326
	½ c	0	tr	tr	94
large					
boiled	½ c	0	tr	tr	108
canned, solids & liquids	½ c	0	tr	tr	95
frozen, boiled, drained	10 oz pkg	0	1	tr	312
	½ c	0	tr	tr	85
long rice *See* mung, *below*					
lupins, boiled	½ c	0	2	tr	98
miso *See* fermented products, *under* SOYBEANS & SOYBEAN PRODUCTS					
moth, boiled	½ c	0	tr	tr	103
mung					
boiled	½ c	0	tr	tr	107
mature seeds, sprouted					
raw	½ c	0	tr	tr	16
	12 oz pkg	0	1	tr	102
boiled, drained	½ c	0	tr	tr	13
canned, drained	½ c	0	tr	tr	8
stir-fried	½ c	0	tr	tr	31
long rice, dehydrated, prepared from mung bean starch	½ c	0	tr	tr	246
mungo, boiled	½ c	0	tr	tr	95
natto *See* fermented products, *under* SOYBEANS & SOYBEAN PRODUCTS					
navy, canned, solids & liq-uids	½ c	0	1	tr	148
okara *See* tofu: okara, *under* SOYBEANS & SOYBEAN PRODUCTS					
pink, boiled	½ c	0	tr	tr	125
pinto					
boiled	½ c	0	tr	tr	117
canned, solids & liquids	½ c	0	tr	tr	93
frozen, boiled, drained	10 oz pkg	0	1	tr	460
Roman *See* cranberry, *above*					
shellie *See* beans, shellie, *under* VEGETABLES, PLAIN & PREPARED					
small white, boiled	½ c	0	1	tr	127
snap *See* beans, snap, *under* VEGETABLES, PLAIN & PREPARED					
soybeans *See* SOYBEANS & SOYBEAN PRODUCTS					

	Portion	Chol (mg)	Total Fat (g)	Satur'd Fat (g)	Total Calor
tempeh *See* fermented products, *under* SOYBEANS & SOYBEAN PRODUCTS					
white					
boiled	½ c	0	tr	tr	125
canned, solids & liquids	½ c	0	tr	tr	153
winged					
raw	½ c	0	15	2	372
boiled	½ c	0	5	1	126
winged bean leaves, raw	3½ oz	0	1	tr	74
winged bean tuber, raw	3½ oz	0	1	tr	159
yardlong					
raw	½ c	0	1	tr	292
boiled	½ c	0	tr	tr	102
yellow, boiled	½ c	0	1	tr	126
yokan *See* adzuki, *above*					

Peas & Lentils

	Portion	Chol (mg)	Total Fat (g)	Satur'd Fat (g)	Total Calor
Bengal gram *See* chickpeas, *below*					
black-eyed *See* cowpeas, common, *below*					
chickpeas					
boiled	½ c	0	2	tr	134
canned, solids & liquids	½ c	0	1	tr	143
cowpeas, catjang, boiled	½ c	0	1	tr	100
cowpeas, common					
boiled	½ c	0	tr	tr	100
canned, plain, solids & liquids	½ c	0	1	tr	92
frozen, boiled, drained	½ c	0	1	tr	112
cowpeas, leafy tips					
raw	1 c	0	tr	tr	10
boiled, drained	½ c	0	tr	tr	6
cowpeas, young pods w/ seeds					
raw	1 pod = 0.4 oz	0	tr	tr	5
boiled, drained	½ c	0	tr	tr	16
crowder peas *See* cowpeas, common, *above*					
golden gram *See* chickpeas, *above*					
lentils					
boiled	½ c	0	tr	tr	115
sprouted					
raw	½ c	0	tr	tr	40
stir-fried	3½ oz	0	tr	tr	101
pigeon peas					
raw	½ c	0	2	tr	350
boiled	½ c	0	tr	tr	102
red gram *See* pigeon peas, *above*					
southern peas *See* cowpeas, common, *above*					
split peas, boiled	½ c	0	tr	tr	116

	Portion	Chol (mg)	Total Fat (g)	Satur'd Fat (g)	Total Calor
Prepared Bean Dishes					
baked beans					
canned					
plain or vegetarian	½ c	0	1	tr	118
w/beef	½ c	29	5	2	161
w/franks	½ c	8	8	3	182
w/pork	½ c	9	2	1	133
w/pork & sweet sauce	½ c	9	2	1	140
w/pork & tomato sauce	½ c	9	1	tr	123
homemade	½ c	6	6	2	190
chili w/beans, canned	½ c	22	7	3	144
cowpeas, common, canned, w/pork	½ c	8	2	1	99
falafel	0.6 oz	0	3	tr	57
	1.8 oz	0	9	1	170
hummus	1 c	0	21	3	420
refried beans, canned	½ c	?	1	1	134
▪ **BRAND NAME**					
Armour Star					
chili					
w/beans	7½ oz	?	26	?	390
w/out beans	7½ oz	?	29	?	380
Texas chili w/beans	7½ oz	?	26	?	370
Arrowhead Mills					
adzuki beans	2 oz	0	1	?	190
anasazi beans	2 oz	0	1	?	200
black turtle beans	2 oz	0	1	?	190
chickpeas	2 oz	0	3	?	200
kidney beans	2 oz	0	1	?	190
lentils					
green	2 oz	0	1	?	190
red	2 oz	0	1	?	195
mung beans					
dry, raw	2 oz	0	?	?	?
sprouted	1 c	0	0	0	50
pinto beans	2 oz	0	1	?	200
split peas, green	2 oz	0	1	?	200
Campbell					
barbecue beans	7⅞ oz	?	4	?	250
Home Style beans	8 oz	?	4	?	270
Old Fashioned beans in molasses & brown sugar	8 oz	?	3	?	270

	Portion	Chol (mg)	Total Fat (g)	Satur'd Fat (g)	Total Calor
pork & beans in tomato sauce	8 oz	?	3	?	240
Ranchero beans	7⅞ oz	?	5	?	220
Fearn					
BEAN MIXES					
bean barley stew	½ of 3½ oz box	tr	2	tr	180
black bean creole	½ of 3¾ oz box	tr	2	tr	180
lentil minestrone soup	½ of 3¾ oz box	tr	1	tr	160
split pea soup	½ of 3½ oz box	tr	3	1	180
tri-bean casserole	½ of 3¼ oz box	tr	2	tr	160
VEGETARIAN MIXES					
breakfast patty	⅛ of 7.4 oz box	0	6	1	110
falafel	⅑ of 7.4 oz box	0	2	tr	80
sesame burger	¼ c dry or ⅛ of 8.4 oz box	0	7	1	130
sunflower burger	¼ c dry or ⅛ of 8.4 oz box	0	4	1	120
Featherweight					
chili w/beans	7½ oz	?	13	?	270
Health Valley					
BEANS					
Boston baked, regular or no salt	4 oz	0	1	?	130
vegetarian, w/miso	4 oz	0	1	?	120
CHILI					
con carne	4 oz	?	8	?	170
mild vegetarian w/beans, regular or no salt	4 oz	0	7	?	170
spicy vegetarian w/beans					
regular	4 oz	0	7	?	170
no salt	4 oz	0	7	?	180
w/lentils, regular or low-sodium	4 oz	0	6	?	120
LENTILS					
Zesty pilaf, regular or no salt	4 oz	0	3	?	110

	Portion	Chol (mg)	Total Fat (g)	Satur'd Fat (g)	Total Calor
Van Camp's					
Beanie Weenee	1 c	?	15	?	326
brown sugar beans	1 c	?	5	?	284
butter beans	1 c	?	1	?	162
chili					
w/beans	1 c	?	23	?	352
w/out beans	1 c	?	34	?	412
kidney beans					
dark red	1 c	?	1	?	182
light red	1 c	?	1	?	184
New Orleans–style red	1 c	?	1	?	178
Mexican-style chili beans	1 c	?	2	?	210
pork & beans	1 c	?	2	?	216
red beans	1 c	?	1	?	194
vegetarian-style beans	1 c	?	1	?	206
Western-style beans	1 c	?	4	?	207
Wolf					
chili w/beans	1 c	?	22	?	345
chili w/out beans					
regular	1 c	?	27	?	387
extra spicy	scant c	?	25	?	363

□ **LUNCHEON MEATS** *See* PROCESSED MEAT & POULTRY PRODUCTS

□ **MAIN COURSES** *See* ENTREES & MAIN COURSES, CANNED & BOXED; ENTREES & MAIN COURSES, FROZEN

□ **MARGARINE** *See* BUTTER & MARGARINE SPREADS

□ **MARMALADE** *See* FRUIT SPREADS

□ **MAYONNAISE** *See* SALAD DRESSINGS, MAYONNAISE, VINEGAR, & DIPS

□ **MEAT** *See* BEEF, FRESH & CURED; LAMB, VEAL, & MISCELLANEOUS MEATS; PORK, FRESH & CURED; PROCESSED MEAT & POULTRY PRODUCTS

	Portion	Chol (mg)	Total Fat (g)	Satur'd Fat (g)	Total Calor

❏ **MEAT PRODUCTS, SIMULATED** *See* **LEGUMES & LEGUME PRODUCTS; NUTS & NUT-BASED BUTTERS, FLOURS, MEALS, MILKS, PASTES, & POWDERS; SOYBEANS & SOYBEAN PRODUCTS**

❏ **MEAT SPREADS** *See* **PROCESSED MEAT & POULTRY PRODUCTS**

❏ **MILK, MILK SUBSTITUTES, & MILK PRODUCTS: CREAM, SOUR CREAM, CREAM SUBSTITUTES, MILK, MILK SUBSTITUTES, WHEY, & YOGURT**

See also Flavored Milk Beverages, *under* BEVERAGES; CHEESE & CHEESE FOODS; DESSERT SAUCES, SYRUPS, & TOPPINGS

Cream & Sour Cream

CREAM

	Portion	Chol (mg)	Total Fat (g)	Satur'd Fat (g)	Total Calor
half & half	1 T	6	2	1	20
	1 c	89	28	17	315
light	1 T	10	3	2	29
	1 c	159	46	29	469
medium (25% fat)	1 T	13	4	2	37
	1 c	209	60	37	583
whipping					
light	1 T	17	5	3	44
	1 c or about 2 c whipped	265	74	46	699
heavy	1 T	21	6	3	52
	1 c or about 2 c whipped	326	88	55	821

SOUR CREAM

	Portion	Chol (mg)	Total Fat (g)	Satur'd Fat (g)	Total Calor
cultured	1 T	5	3	2	26
	1 c	102	48	30	493
half & half, cultured	1 T	6	2	1	20

	Portion	Chol (mg)	Total Fat (g)	Satur'd Fat (g)	Total Calor
Cream & Sour Cream Substitutes					
coffee whitener, nondairy					
liquid, frozen	½ fl oz	0	2	tr	20
	½ c	0	12	2	163
liquid, frozen, containing lauric acid oil & sodium caseinate	½ fl oz	0	2	1	20
	½ c	0	12	11	164
powdered, containing lauric acid oil & sodium caseinate	1 t	0	1	1	11
imitation sour cream, non-dairy, cultured, containing lauric acid oil & sodium caseinate	1 oz	0	6	5	59
	1 c	0	45	41	479
sour dressing, nonbutter-fat, cultured (made by combining fats or oils other than milk fat w/ milk solids)	1 T	1	2	2	21
	1 c	13	39	31	417

Milk, Cows'

FRESH

whole					
3.7% fat, pasteurized or raw	1 c	35	9	6	157
low-sodium	1 c	33	8	5	149
low-fat					
2% fat	1 c	18	5	3	121
2% fat, nonfat milk solids added	1 c	18	5	3	125
2% fat, protein-fortified	1 c	19	5	3	137
1% fat	1 c	10	3	2	102
1% fat, nonfat milk solids added	1 c	10	2	1	104
1% fat, protein-fortified	1 c	10	3	2	119
skim	1 c	4	tr	tr	86
skim, nonfat milk solids added	1 c	5	1	tr	90
skim, protein-fortified	1 c	5	1	tr	100
buttermilk, cultured	1 c	9	2	1	99

CONDENSED & EVAPORATED

condensed, sweetened, canned	1 oz	13	3	2	123
	1 c	104	27	17	982
evaporated, canned					
whole	1 oz	9	2	1	42
	½ c	37	10	6	169
skim	1 fl oz	1	tr	tr	25
	½ c	5	tr	tr	99

	Portion	Chol (mg)	Total Fat (g)	Satur'd Fat (g)	Total Calor
DRY					
whole	¼ c	31	9	5	159
	1 c	124	34	21	635
nonfat					
regular	¼ c	6	tr	tr	109
	1 c	24	1	1	435
calcium-reduced	1 oz	1	tr	tr	100
instant	3.2 oz	17	1	tr	326
	1 c	12	tr	tr	244
buttermilk, sweet cream	1 T	5	tr	tr	25
	1 c	83	7	4	464

Milk, Other

goat	1 c	28	10	7	168
human	1 oz	4	1	1	21
Indian buffalo	1 c	46	17	11	236
sheep	1 c	?	17	11	264

Milk Substitutes

filled (made by blending hydrogenated vegetable oils w/milk solids)	1 c	4	8	2	154
filled, w/lauric acid oil (made by combining milk solids w/fats or oils other than milk fat)	1 c	4	8	8	153
imitation, containing blend of hydrogenated vegetable oils	1 c	tr	8	2	150
imitation, containing lauric acid	1 c	tr	8	7	150

Whey

acid					
dry	1 T	?	tr	tr	10
fluid	1 c	?	tr	tr	59
sweet					
dry	1 T	tr	tr	tr	26
fluid	1 c	5	1	1	66

Yogurt

plain					
8 g protein	1 c	29	7	5	139
low-fat, 12 g protein	1 c	14	4	2	144
skim milk, 13 g protein	1 c	4	tr	tr	127

	Portion	Chol (mg)	Total Fat (g)	Satur'd Fat (g)	Total Calor
coffee & vanilla varieties, low-fat, 11 g protein	1 c	11	3	2	194
fruit varieties, low-fat					
9 g protein	1 c	10	3	2	225
10 g protein	1 c	10	2	2	231
11 g protein	1 c	12	3	2	239

▪ BRAND NAME

Colombo Yogurt
LITE

	Portion	Chol (mg)	Total Fat (g)	Satur'd Fat (g)	Total Calor
plain	8 oz	0	0	?	110
strawberry	8 oz	0	0	?	200
vanilla	8 oz	0	0	?	160

WHOLE MILK

	Portion	Chol (mg)	Total Fat (g)	Satur'd Fat (g)	Total Calor
plain	8 oz	23	7	?	150
banana strawberry	8 oz	18	6	?	235
blueberry	8 oz	18	7	?	250
French vanilla	8 oz	18	7	?	210
peach	8 oz	18	6	?	230
strawberry	8 oz	18	6	?	230
strawberry vanilla	8 oz	18	6	?	260

Friendship

	Portion	Chol (mg)	Total Fat (g)	Satur'd Fat (g)	Total Calor
buttermilk, low-fat (1½% milk fat)	1 c	14	4	?	120
Lite Delite low-fat sour cream	2 T	8	2	?	35
sour cream	2 T	42	5	?	55
yogurt					
regular (3½% milk fat), plain	1 c	30	8	?	170
low-fat (1½% milk fat)					
vanilla & coffee	1 c	14	3	?	210
w/fruit	1 c	14	3	?	230

Land O'Lakes

	Portion	Chol (mg)	Total Fat (g)	Satur'd Fat (g)	Total Calor
buttermilk	8 fl oz	10	2	1	100
Flash instant, nonfat, re-constituted dry milk	8 fl oz	5	<1	<1	80
Gourmet heavy whipping cream	1 T	20	6	4	60
half & half	1 T	5	2	1	20
milk					
homogenized	8 fl oz	35	8	5	150
low-fat (2%)	8 fl oz	20	5	3	120
low-fat (1%)	8 fl oz	10	3	2	100
skim	8 fl oz	5	<1	<1	90
sour cream	1 T	5	3	2	25
whipping cream	1 T	15	5	3	45

	Portion	Chol (mg)	Total Fat (g)	Satur'd Fat (g)	Total Calor
La Yogurt					
plain	6 oz	?	3	?	130
Rich's Nondairy Creamers					
Coffee Rich	½ oz	0	2	tr	22
Poly Rich	½ oz	0	1	tr	22
Richwhip					
liquid	¼ oz or 1 fl oz whipped	0	2	1	20
pressurized	¼ oz	0	2	1	20
prewhipped	1 T whipped	0	1	1	12
Whitney's Yogurt					
plain	6 oz	?	7	?	150
apples & raisins	6 oz	?	5	?	200
blueberry	6 oz	?	5	?	200
boysenberry	6 oz	?	5	?	200
cherry	6 oz	?	5	?	200
coffee	6 oz	?	6	?	200
lemon	6 oz	?	6	?	200
peach	6 oz	?	5	?	200
piña colada	6 oz	?	7	?	210
raspberry	6 oz	?	5	?	200
strawberry	6 oz	?	5	?	200
strawberry banana	6 oz	?	5	?	200
tropical fruits	6 oz	?	6	?	200
vanilla	6 oz	?	6	?	200
wild berries	6 oz	?	5	?	200

❑ MOLASSES *See* SUGARS & SWEETENERS

❑ MUFFINS *See* BREADS, ROLLS, BISCUITS, & MUFFINS

❑ NOODLES & PASTA, PLAIN

Noodles

chow funn, dry (Oriental wheat noodles)	1 oz	0	tr	?	102
chow mein, canned	1 c	5	11	2	220
egg, enriched, cooked	1 c	50	2	1	200

Japanese style, seasoned *See* Nissin, *under* SOUPS, PREPARED

	Portion	Chol (mg)	Total Fat (g)	Satur'd Fat (g)	Total Calor
rice, dry	1 oz	0	1	?	130
saimin, dry (Oriental wheat noodles)	1 oz	0	0	?	95
soba, dry (Oriental buck-wheat noodles)	1 oz	0	1	?	99

Pasta

	Portion	Chol (mg)	Total Fat (g)	Satur'd Fat (g)	Total Calor
macaroni, enriched, cooked (cut lengths, elbows, shells)					
firm stage, hot	1 c	0	1	tr	190
tender stage					
cold	1 c	0	tr	tr	115
hot	1 c	0	1	tr	155

prepared & seasoned pasta dishes *See* DINNERS, FROZEN; ENTREES & MAIN COURSES, CANNED & BOXED; ENTREES & MAIN COURSES, FROZEN

	Portion	Chol (mg)	Total Fat (g)	Satur'd Fat (g)	Total Calor
spaghetti, enriched, cooked					
firm stage, hot	1 c	0	1	tr	190
tender stage, hot	1 c	0	1	tr	155

▪ BRAND NAME

Health Valley

	Portion	Chol (mg)	Total Fat (g)	Satur'd Fat (g)	Total Calor
elbows, whole-wheat or whole-wheat w/4 vegetables	2 oz dry	0	1	?	202
lasagna, whole-wheat	2 oz dry	0	1	?	200
spaghetti: whole-wheat, whole-wheat amaranth, or whole-wheat w/spinach	2 oz dry	0	1	?	200
spinach lasagna, whole-wheat	2 oz dry	0	1	?	170

Mueller's

	Portion	Chol (mg)	Total Fat (g)	Satur'd Fat (g)	Total Calor
egg noodles	2 oz dry	55	3	?	220
Golden Rich egg noodles	2 oz dry	70	3	?	220
lasagna	2 oz dry	0	1	?	210
spaghetti & macaroni	2 oz dry	0	1	?	210
tricolor twists	2 oz dry	0	1	?	210

Prince

	Portion	Chol (mg)	Total Fat (g)	Satur'd Fat (g)	Total Calor
egg noodles	3½ oz dry	65	3	?	380
macaroni & spaghetti	3½ oz dry	0	2	?	370
Superoni	3½ oz dry	0	0	?	360

	Portion	Chol (mg)	Total Fat (g)	Satur'd Fat (g)	Total Calor

❑ NUTS & NUT-BASED BUTTERS, FLOURS, MEALS, MILKS, PASTES, & POWDERS

See also SEEDS & SEED-BASED BUTTERS, FLOURS, & MEALS

	Portion	Chol (mg)	Total Fat (g)	Satur'd Fat (g)	Total Calor
acorn flour, full-fat	1 oz	0	9	1	142
acorns					
raw	1 oz	0	7	1	105
dried	1 oz	0	9	1	145
almond butter					
plain	1 T	0	9	1	101
honey & cinnamon	1 T	0	8	1	96
almond meal, partially de-fatted	1 oz	0	5	tr	116
almond paste	1 oz	0	8	1	127
	1 c firmly packed	0	62	6	1,012
almond powder					
full-fat	1 oz	0	15	1	168
	1 c not packed	0	34	3	385
partially defatted	1 oz	0	5	tr	112
	1 c not packed	0	10	1	255
almonds					
dried					
blanched	1 oz	0	15	1	166
	1 c whole kernels	0	76	7	850
unblanched	1 oz	0	15	1	167
	1 c whole kernels	0	74	7	837
dry roasted, unblanched	1 oz	0	15	1	167
	1 c whole kernels	0	71	7	810
oil roasted					
blanched	1 oz	0	16	2	174
	1 c whole kernels	0	80	8	870
unblanched	1 oz	0	16	2	176
	1 c whole kernels	0	91	9	970
toasted, unblanched	1 oz	0	14	1	167
beechnuts, dried	1 oz	0	14	2	164
Brazil nuts, dried, un-blanched	1 oz	0	19	5	186
	1 c	0	93	23	919
butternuts, dried	1 oz	0	16	tr	174
cashew butter, plain	1 T	0	8	2	94

	Portion	Chol (mg)	Total Fat (g)	Satur'd Fat (g)	Total Calor
cashew nuts					
dry roasted	1 oz	0	13	3	163
	1 c wholes & halves	0	64	13	787
oil roasted	1 oz	0	14	3	163
	1 c wholes & halves	0	63	12	748
chestnuts, Chinese					
raw	1 oz	0	tr	tr	64
boiled, steamed	1 oz	0	tr	tr	44
dried	1 oz	0	1	tr	103
roasted	1 oz	0	tr	tr	68
chestnuts, European raw					
peeled	1 oz	0	tr	tr	56
unpeeled	1 oz	0	1	tr	60
	1 c	0	3	1	308
boiled, steamed	1 oz	0	tr	tr	37
dried					
peeled	1 oz	0	1	tr	105
unpeeled	1 oz	0	1	tr	106
roasted	1 oz	0	1	tr	70
	1 c	0	3	1	350
chestnuts, Japanese					
raw	1 oz	0	tr	tr	44
boiled, steamed	1 oz	0	tr	tr	16
dried	1 oz	0	tr	tr	102
	1 c	0	2	tr	558
roasted	1 oz	0	tr	tr	57
coconut cream					
raw	1 T	0	5	5	49
	1 c	0	83	74	792
canned	1 T	0	3	3	36
	1 c	0	52	47	568
coconut meat					
raw	1.6 oz	0	15	13	159
	1 c shredded or grated	0	27	24	283
dried (desiccated)					
creamed	1 oz	0	20	17	194
sweetened, flaked, canned	4 oz	0	36	32	505
	1 c	0	24	22	341
sweetened, flaked, packaged	7 oz	0	64	57	944
	1 c	0	24	21	351
sweetened, shredded	7 oz	0	71	63	997
	1 c	0	33	29	466
toasted	1 oz	0	13	12	168
unsweetened	1 oz	0	18	16	187
coconut milk					
raw	1 T	0	4	3	35
	1 c	0	57	51	552

	Portion	Chol (mg)	Total Fat (g)	Satur'd Fat (g)	Total Calor
canned	1 T	0	3	3	30
	1 c	0	48	43	445
frozen	1 T	0	3	3	30
	1 c	0	50	44	486
coconut water	1 T	0	tr	tr	3
	1 c	0	tr	tr	46
filberts or hazelnuts dried					
blanched	1 oz	0	19	1	191
unblanched	1 oz	0	18	1	179
	1 c chopped kernels	0	72	5	727
dry roasted, unblanched	1 oz	0	19	1	188
oil roasted, unblanched	1 oz	0	18	1	187
formulated nuts, wheat-based					
unflavored	1 oz	0	16	2	177
macadamia-flavored	1 oz	0	16	2	176
all other flavors	1 oz	0	18	3	184
ginkgo nuts					
raw	1 oz	0	tr	tr	52
canned	1 oz	0	tr	tr	32
	1 c	0	3	tr	173
dried	1 oz	0	1	tr	99
hazelnuts *See* filberts, *above*					
hickory nuts, dried	1 oz	0	18	2	187
macadamia nuts					
dried	1 oz	0	21	3	199
	1 c	0	99	15	940
oil roasted	1 oz	0	22	3	204
	1 c wholes or halves	0	103	15	962
mixed nuts (cashew nuts, almonds, filberts, & pecans)					
dry roasted, w/peanuts	1 oz	0	15	2	169
	1 c	0	70	9	814
oil roasted					
w/peanuts	1 oz	0	16	2	175
	1 c	0	80	12	876
w/out peanuts	1 oz	0	16	3	175
	1 c	0	81	13	886
peanut butter, w/added fat, sugar, & salt, chunk or smooth style	2 T	0	16	3	188
peanut flour					
defatted	1 T	0	tr	tr	13
	1 c	0	tr	tr	196
low-fat	1 c	?	13	2	257

	Portion	Chol (mg)	Total Fat (g)	Satur'd Fat (g)	Total Calor
peanuts					
all types					
raw	1 oz	0	14	2	159
	1 c	0	72	10	828
boiled	½ c	0	7	1	102
dried	1 oz	0	14	2	161
	1 c	0	72	10	827
dry roasted	1 oz	0	14	2	164
	1 c	0	73	10	855
oil roasted	1 oz	0	14	2	163
	1 c	0	71	10	837
Spanish, oil roasted	1 oz	0	14	2	162
	1 c	0	72	11	851
Valencia, oil roasted	1 oz	0	14	2	165
	1 c	0	74	11	848
Virginia, oil roasted	1 oz	0	14	2	161
	1 c	0	70	9	826
pecan flour	1 oz	0	tr	tr	93
pecans					
dried	1 oz	0	19	2	190
	1 c halves	0	73	6	721
dry roasted	1 oz	0	18	1	187
oil roasted	1 oz	0	20	2	195
	1 c	0	78	6	754
pignolias *See* pine nuts, *below*					
pili nuts, dried	1 oz	0	23	9	204
	1 c	0	95	37	863
pine nuts					
pignolia, dried	1 oz	0	14	2	146
	1 T	0	5	1	51
piñon, dried	1 oz	0	17	3	161
	10 kernels	0	1	tr	6
pistachios					
dried	1 oz	0	14	2	164
	1 c	0	62	8	739
dry roasted	1 oz	0	15	2	172
	1 c	0	68	9	776
sweet chestnuts *See* chestnuts, European, *above*					
walnuts					
black, dried	1 oz	0	16	1	172
	1 c chopped	0	71	5	759
English or Persian, dried	1 oz	0	18	2	182
	1 c pieces	0	74	7	770

▪ BRAND NAME

Arrowhead Mills

peanut butter, creamy or chunky	2 T	0	16	?	190

	Portion	Chol (mg)	Total Fat (g)	Satur'd Fat (g)	Total Calor
Blue Diamond					
almonds					
raw, whole, unblanched	1 oz	0	14	1	173
blanched, sliced	1 oz	0	15	?	176
blanched, whole, raw	1 oz	0	14	2	174
dry roasted, unsalted	1 oz	0	15	?	168
oil roasted, salted	1 oz	0	16	?	174
hazelnuts					
raw, whole, Oregon	1 oz	0	15	1	166
oil roasted, salted	1 oz	0	18	?	180
macadamia nuts, dry roasted, salted	1 oz	0	21	3	193
pistachios, dry roasted, salted, natural, California	1 oz	0	14	2	162
Erewhon					
almond butter	1 T	0	8	?	90
peanut butter, chunky or creamy, salted or un- salted	2 T	0	14	?	190
Fearn					
Brazil nut burger mix	¼ c dry or ⅛ of 7.6 oz box	0	4	1	100
Featherweight					
low-sodium peanut butter					
chunky	1 oz	?	7	?	90
creamy	1 oz	?	15	?	180
Planters					
almonds					
blanched: slivered, whole, or sliced	1 oz	0	15	2	170
dry roasted	1 oz	0	15	2	170
honey roasted	1 oz	0	13	1	170
cashews					
dry roasted, regular or unsalted	1 oz	0	13	3	230
honey roasted	1 oz	0	12	2	170
oil roasted, fancy or halves, regular or un- salted	1 oz	0	14	3	170
cashews & peanuts, honey roasted	1 oz	0	12	2	170
mixed nuts					
dry roasted					
regular	1 oz	0	14	2	160
unsalted	1 oz	0	15	2	170
oil roasted					
deluxe	1 oz	0	17	3	180
regular or unsalted	1 oz	0	16	3	180

	Portion	Chol (mg)	Total Fat (g)	Satur'd Fat (g)	Total Calor
nut topping	1 oz	0	16	2	180
peanuts					
cocktail, oil roasted, regular or unsalted	1 oz	0	15	3	170
dry roasted					
regular	1 oz	0	14	2	160
unsalted	1 oz	0	15	2	170
honey roasted					
regular	1 oz	0	13	2	170
dry roasted	1 oz	0	13	2	160
oil roasted, salted	1 oz	0	15	3	170
redskin, oil roasted	1 oz	0	15	5	170
roasted-in-shell, salted or unsalted	1 oz	0	14	2	160
Spanish					
raw	1 oz	0	12	2	150
dry roasted	1 oz	0	14	3	160
oil roasted	1 oz	0	15	5	170
Sweet 'n Crunchy	1 oz	0	8	1	140
pecans: chips, halves, or pieces	1 oz	0	20	2	190
pistachios					
dry roasted	1 oz	0	15	2	170
natural	1 oz	0	5	2	170
red	1 oz	0	15	2	170
sesame nut mix					
dry roasted	1 oz	0	12	3	160
oil roasted	1 oz	0	13	2	160
sunflower nuts					
dry roasted					
regular	1 oz	0	14	2	160
unsalted	1 oz	0	15	2	170
oil roasted	1 oz	0	15	4	170
Tavern Nuts	1 oz	0	15	2	170
walnuts					
black	1 oz	0	17	1	180
English: whole, halves, or pieces	1 oz	0	20	2	190
Skippy Peanut Butter					
creamy or super chunk	2 T	0	17	3	190
	1 T	0	8	2	95
Smucker's					
natural peanut butter	2 T	0	16	1	200

❑ **OILS** *See* FATS, OILS, & SHORTENINGS

	Portion	Chol (mg)	Total Fat (g)	Satur'd Fat (g)	Total Calor

☐ **OLIVES** *See* **PICKLES, OLIVES, RELISHES, & CHUTNEYS**

☐ **PASTA** *See* **NOODLES & PASTA, PLAIN**

☐ **PASTRIES** *See* **DESSERTS: CAKES, PASTRIES, & PIES**

☐ **PÂTÉS** *See* **PROCESSED MEAT & POULTRY PRODUCTS**

☐ **PEANUT BUTTER** *See* **NUTS & NUT-BASED BUTTERS, FLOURS, MEALS, MILKS, PASTES, & POWDERS**

☐ **PICKLES, OLIVES, RELISHES, & CHUTNEYS**
See also peppers; sauerkraut, *under* VEGETABLES, PLAIN & PREPARED

Chutneys

	Portion	Chol (mg)	Total Fat (g)	Satur'd Fat (g)	Total Calor
apple	1 T	0	tr	?	41
tomato	1 T	0	?	?	31

Olives, Canned

	Portion	Chol (mg)	Total Fat (g)	Satur'd Fat (g)	Total Calor
green	4 medium or 3 extra large	0	2	tr	15
ripe, Mission, pitted	3 small or 2 large	0	2	tr	15

Pickles, Cucumber

	Portion	Chol (mg)	Total Fat (g)	Satur'd Fat (g)	Total Calor
bread & butter	4 slices	0	tr	?	18
dill, whole	1 medium = about 2¼ oz	0	tr	tr	5

	Portion	Chol (mg)	Total Fat (g)	Satur'd Fat (g)	Total Calor
fresh-pack	2 slices = about ½ oz	0	tr	tr	10
kosher	1	0	tr	tr	7
sour	1 large	0	tr	tr	10
sweet	1 large	0	tr	tr	146
sweet & sour, sliced	1 slice	0	tr	tr	3
sweet gherkin, small, whole	1 = about ½ oz	0	tr	tr	20

Relishes

cranberry-orange	1 T	0	tr	?	27
canned	½ c	0	tr	?	246
pickle					
chow chow					
sour	1 oz	0	tr	tr	8
sweet	1 oz	0	tr	?	32
sour	1 T	0	tr	?	3
sweet, finely chopped	1 T	0	tr	tr	20
strawberry	1 T	0	0	0	53
strawberry-pineapple	1 T	0	0	0	54
tomato	1 T	0	tr	?	53

▪ BRAND NAME

Claussen					
kosher tomatoes	1	0	tr	tr	5
pickled cucumbers	1	0	0 or tr	0 or tr	varies
Dromedary					
pimientos, all types, drained	1 oz	?	0	?	10
Vlasic					
pickled cucumbers, onions, peppers	1 oz	0	0	0	varies
relishes, hamburger & hot dog	1 oz	0	0	0	varies

❑ PIE FILLINGS *See* DESSERTS: CUSTARDS, GELATINS, PUDDINGS, & PIE FILLINGS

❑ PIES *See* DESSERTS: CAKES, PASTRIES, & PIES

	Portion	Chol (mg)	Total Fat (g)	Satur'd Fat (g)	Total Calor
PIZZA					
pizza, cheese	⅛ pizza (15" diam)	56	9	4	290
BRAND NAME					
Celentano					
9-slice pizza	⅑ pizza = 2.67 oz	?	5	?	157
thick crust pizza	⅓ pizza = 4.3 oz	?	7	?	238
Celeste Frozen Pizza					
Canadian-style bacon	7¾ oz pizza	?	26	?	541
	¼ of 19 oz pizza	?	17	?	329
cheese	6½ oz pizza	?	25	?	497
	¼ of 17¾ oz pizza	?	17	?	317
deluxe	8¼ oz pizza	?	32	?	582
	¼ of 22¼ oz pizza	?	22	?	378
pepperoni	6¾ oz pizza	?	30	?	546
	¼ of 19 oz pizza	?	21	?	368
sausage	7½ oz pizza	?	32	?	571
	¼ of 20 oz pizza	?	22	?	376
sausage & mushroom	8½ oz pizza	?	32	?	592
	¼ of 22½ oz pizza	?	22	?	387
Suprema	9 oz pizza	?	39	?	678
	¼ of 23 oz pizza	?	24	?	381
Pepperidge Farm Croissant Pastry Pizza					
cheese	1	?	27	?	490
deluxe	1	?	27	?	520
hamburger	1	?	27	?	510
pepperoni	1	?	25	?	490
sausage	1	?	29	?	540

	Portion	Chol (mg)	Total Fat (g)	Satur'd Fat (g)	Total Calor
Stouffer's French Bread Frozen Pizza					
cheese	½ pkg	?	13	?	340
deluxe	½ pkg	?	21	?	430
hamburger	½ pkg	?	18	?	410
pepperoni	½ pkg	?	18	?	390
sausage	½ pkg	?	20	?	420
sausage & mushroom	½ pkg	?	17	?	400

❑ PORK, FRESH & CURED
See also PROCESSED MEAT & POULTRY PRODUCTS

Pork, Fresh

	Portion	Chol (mg)	Total Fat (g)	Satur'd Fat (g)	Total Calor
retail cuts, separable fat, cooked	1 oz	26	21	8	200
LEG (HAM)					
Lean & Fat					
whole, roasted	3 oz	79	18	6	250
	1 c	131	29	11	411
rump half, roasted	3 oz	81	15	5	233
	1 c	133	25	9	384
shank half, roasted	3 oz	78	19	7	258
	1 c	129	31	11	425
Lean Only					
whole, roasted	3 oz	80	9	3	187
	1 c	131	15	5	309
rump half, roasted	3 oz	81	9	3	187
	1 c	134	15	5	309
shank half, roasted	3 oz	78	9	3	183
	1 c	129	15	5	301
LOIN, WHOLE					
Lean & Fat					
braised	3 oz	87	24	9	312
	1 chop (3 chops/lb as pur-chased)	73	20	7	261
broiled	3 oz	80	23	8	294
	1 chop (3 chops/lb as pur-chased)	77	22	8	284

	Portion	Chol (mg)	Total Fat (g)	Satur'd Fat (g)	Total Calor
roasted	3 oz	77	21	7	271
	1 chop (3 chops/lb as purchased)	74	20	7	262
Lean Only					
braised	3 oz	90	12	4	232
	1 chop (3 chops/lb as purchased)	58	8	3	150
broiled	3 oz	81	13	4	218
	1 chop (3 chops/lb as purchased)	63	10	3	169
roasted	3 oz	77	12	4	204
	1 chop (3 chops/lb as purchased)	62	10	3	166
LOIN, BLADE					
Lean & Fat					
braised	3 oz	92	29	10	348
	1 chop (3 chops/lb as purchased)	72	23	8	275
broiled	3 oz	83	29	10	334
	1 chop (3 chops/lb as purchased)	75	26	9	303
pan-fried	3 oz	81	31	11	352
	1 chop (3 chops/lb as purchased)	85	33	12	368
roasted	3 oz	76	26	9	310
	1 chop (3 chops/lb as purchased)	79	27	10	321

	Portion	Chol (mg)	Total Fat (g)	Satur'd Fat (g)	Total Calor
Lean Only					
braised	3 oz	96	18	6	266
	1 chop (3 chops/lb as pur- chased)	57	10	4	156
broiled	3 oz	85	18	6	255
	1 chop (3 chops/lb as pur- chased)	59	13	4	177
pan-fried	3 oz	82	17	6	240
	1 chop (3 chops/lb as pur- chased)	60	12	4	175
roasted	3 oz	76	16	6	238
	1 chop (3 chops/lb as pur- chased)	63	14	5	198
LOIN, CENTER					
Lean & Fat					
braised	3 oz	91	22	8	301
	1 chop (3 chops/lb as pur- chased)	81	19	7	266
broiled	3 oz	82	19	7	269
	1 chop (3 chops/lb as pur- chased)	84	19	7	275
pan-fried	3 oz	87	26	9	318
	1 chop (3 chops/lb as pur- chased)	92	27	10	333
roasted	3 oz	78	18	7	259
	1 chop (3 chops/lb as pur- chased)	80	19	7	268

	Portion	Chol (mg)	Total Fat (g)	Satur'd Fat (g)	Total Calor
Lean Only					
braised	3 oz	95	12	4	231
	1 chop (3 chops/lb as pur- chased)	68	8	3	166
broiled	3 oz	83	9	3	196
	1 chop (3 chops/lb as pur- chased)	71	8	3	166
pan-fried	3 oz	91	14	5	226
	1 chop (3 chops/lb as pur- chased)	71	11	4	178
roasted	3 oz	78	11	4	204
	1 chop (3 chops/lb as pur- chased)	68	10	3	180
LOIN, CENTER RIB					
Lean & Fat					
braised	3 oz	81	23	8	312
	1 chop (3 chops/lb as pur- chased)	64	18	7	246
broiled	3 oz	79	22	8	291
	1 chop (3 chops/lb as pur- chased)	72	20	7	264
pan-fried	3 oz	71	28	10	331
	1 chop (3 chops/lb as pur- chased)	74	29	10	343
roasted	3 oz	69	20	7	271
	1 chop (3 chops/lb as pur- chased)	64	19	7	252

	Portion	Chol (mg)	Total Fat (g)	Satur'd Fat (g)	Total Calor
Lean Only					
braised	3 oz	82	12	4	236
	1 chop (3 chops/lb as purchased)	51	8	3	147
broiled	3 oz	80	13	4	219
	1 chop (3 chops/lb as purchased)	59	9	3	162
pan-fried	3 oz	69	13	4	219
	1 chop (3 chops/lb as purchased)	50	9	3	160
roasted	3 oz	67	12	4	208
	1 chop (3 chops/lb as purchased)	52	9	3	162
LOIN, SIRLOIN					
Lean & Fat					
braised	3 oz	90	22	8	299
	1 chop (3 chops/lb as purchased)	75	18	7	250
broiled	3 oz	82	21	8	281
	1 chop (3 chops/lb as purchased)	81	21	8	278
roasted	3 oz	77	17	6	247
	1 chop (3 chops/lb as purchased)	76	17	6	244

	Portion	Chol (mg)	Total Fat (g)	Satur'd Fat (g)	Total Calor
Lean Only					
braised	3 oz	94	11	4	221
	1 chop (3 chops/lb as pur- chased)	63	7	3	149
broiled	3 oz	83	12	4	207
	1 chop (3 chops/lb as pur- chased)	67	9	3	165
roasted	3 oz	77	11	4	201
	1 chop (3 chops/lb as pur- chased)	67	10	3	175
LOIN, TENDERLOIN					
lean, roasted	3 oz	79	4	1	141
LOIN, TOP					
Lean & Fat					
braised	3 oz	81	25	9	324
	1 chop (3 chops/lb as pur- chased)	67	20	7	267
broiled	3 oz	79	24	9	306
	1 chop (3 chops/lb as pur- chased)	76	23	8	295
pan-fried	3 oz	71	28	10	333
	1 chop (3 chops/lb as pur- chased)	72	29	10	337
roasted	3 oz	69	21	8	280
	1 chop (3 chops/lb as pur- chased)	68	21	8	274

	Portion	Chol (mg)	Total Fat (g)	Satur'd Fat (g)	Total Calor
Lean Only					
braised	3 oz	82	12	4	236
	1 chop (3 chops/lb as pur-chased)	51	8	3	147
broiled	3 oz	80	13	4	219
	1 chop (3 chops/lb as pur-chased)	60	10	3	165
pan-fried	3 oz	69	13	4	219
	1 chop (3 chops/lb as pur-chased)	49	9	3	157
roasted	3 oz	67	12	4	208
	1 chop (3 chops/lb as pur-chased)	54	9	3	167
SHOULDER, WHOLE					
lean & fat, roasted	3 oz	81	22	8	277
	1 c	134	36	13	456
lean only, roasted	3 oz	82	13	4	207
	1 c	135	21	7	341
SHOULDER, ARM PICNIC					
Lean & Fat					
braised	3 oz	93	22	8	293
	1 c	153	36	13	483
roasted	3 oz	80	22	8	281
	1 c	132	37	13	463
Lean Only					
braised	3 oz	97	10	4	211
	1 c	160	17	6	347
roasted	3 oz	81	11	4	194
	1 c	133	18	6	319
SHOULDER, BLADE, BOSTON					
Lean & Fat					
braised	3 oz	95	24	9	316
	1 steak	178	46	17	594
broiled	3 oz	87	24	9	297
	1 steak	190	53	19	647
roasted	3 oz	82	21	8	273
	1 steak	179	47	17	594

	Portion	Chol (mg)	Total Fat (g)	Satur'd Fat (g)	Total Calor
Lean Only					
braised	3 oz	99	15	5	250
	1 steak	151	23	8	382
broiled	3 oz	89	16	5	233
	1 steak	159	28	10	413
roasted	3 oz	83	14	5	218
	1 steak	155	27	9	404
SPARERIBS					
lean & fat, braised	3 oz	103	26	10	338
	6¼ oz (yield from 1 lb as pur- chased)	214	54	21	703
VARIETY MEATS					
brains, braised	3 oz	2,169	8	2	117
chitterlings, simmered	3 oz	122	24	9	258
ears, simmered	1	99	12	?	183
feet, simmered	2½ oz	71	9	3	138
heart, braised	1	285	7	2	191
kidneys, braised	1 c	673	7	2	211
liver, braised	3 oz	302	4	1	141
lungs, braised	3 oz	329	3	1	84
tail, simmered	3 oz	110	30	11	336
tongue, braised	3 oz	124	16	5	230

Pork, Cured

	Portion	Chol (mg)	Total Fat (g)	Satur'd Fat (g)	Total Calor
bacon, pan-fried or roasted	3 medium slices (20 slices/lb)	16	9	3	109
breakfast strips, cooked	3 slices (15 slices/12 oz)	36	12	4	156
	6 oz	179	62	22	780
Canadian-style bacon, un- heated, fully cooked as purchased	2 oz	28	4	1	89
feet, pickled	1 oz	26	5	2	58
ham, boneless regular (about 11% fat)					
unheated	1 oz	16	3	1	52
	1 c	80	15	5	255
roasted	3 oz	50	8	3	151
	1 c	83	13	4	249

	Portion	Chol (mg)	Total Fat (g)	Satur'd Fat (g)	Total Calor
ham, boneless *(cont.)*					
extra lean (about 5% fat)					
unheated	1 oz	13	1	tr	37
	1 c	66	7	2	183
roasted	3 oz	45	5	2	123
	1 c	74	8	3	203
ham, canned					
regular (about 13% fat)					
unheated	1 oz	11	4	1	54
	1 c	55	18	6	266
roasted	3 oz	52	13	4	192
	1 c	86	21	7	317
extra lean (about 4% fat)					
unheated	1 oz	11	1	tr	34
	1 c	53	6	2	168
roasted	3 oz	25	4	1	116
	1 c	41	7	2	191
ham, center slice					
country style, lean only,	4 oz	?	9	3	220
raw	1 oz	?	2	1	55
lean & fat, unheated,	4 oz	61	15	5	229
fully cooked as pur-chased	1 oz	15	4	1	57
ham patties					
unheated, fully cooked as purchased	2.3 oz	46	18	7	206
grilled	2 oz	43	18	7	203
ham steak, boneless, extra lean, unheated, fully cooked as purchased	2 oz	26	2	1	69
ham, whole					
lean & fat					
unheated, fully cooked	1 oz	16	5	2	70
as purchased	1 c	78	26	9	345
roasted	3 oz	52	14	5	207
	1 c	86	23	8	341
lean only					
unheated, fully cooked	1 oz	15	2	1	42
as purchased	1 c	73	8	3	206
roasted	3 oz	47	5	2	133
	1 c	78	8	3	219
salt pork, raw	1 oz	25	23	8	212
separable fat (from ham & arm picnic)					
unheated, fully cooked as purchased	1 oz	19	17	6	164
roasted	1 oz	24	18	6	167
shoulder					
arm picnic, roasted					
lean & fat	3 oz	49	18	7	238
	1 c	82	30	11	392

	Portion	Chol (mg)	Total Fat (g)	Satur'd Fat (g)	Total Calor
lean only	3 oz	41	6	2	145
	1 c	68	10	3	238
blade roll, lean & fat					
unheated, fully cooked as purchased	1 oz	15	6	2	76
roasted	3 oz	57	20	7	244

▪ BRAND NAME

Armour & Armour Star
BACON

	Portion	Chol (mg)	Total Fat (g)	Satur'd Fat (g)	Total Calor
1877 Canadian bacon	2 oz	40	4	?	80
lower salt bacon					
raw	1 slice = 0.3 oz	6	3	?	38
cooked	1 slice = 0.2 oz	5	3	?	30
sliced bacon	1 slice = 0.9 oz	20	13	?	130
thick-sliced bacon	1 slice = 1.3 oz	30	19	?	190

HAM

	Portion	Chol (mg)	Total Fat (g)	Satur'd Fat (g)	Total Calor
boneless, cooked, lower salt, 93% fat-free	1 oz	14	1	?	35
canned	3 oz	50	6	?	120
canned, chopped	3 oz	50	21	?	260
Golden Star, canned	3 oz	50	3	?	90
Speedy Cut, boneless, cooked	1 oz	15	3	?	44

Oscar Mayer
BACON & BREAKFAST STRIPS

	Portion	Chol (mg)	Total Fat (g)	Satur'd Fat (g)	Total Calor
bacon	1 cooked slice	5	3	1	35
Bacon Bits	¼ oz	6	1	tr	21
breakfast strips	1 strip, raw	14	5	2	52
Canadian-style bacon	1 oz	12	1	1	35
thick-sliced bacon	1 cooked slice	10	6	2	64

HAM

	Portion	Chol (mg)	Total Fat (g)	Satur'd Fat (g)	Total Calor
boneless Jubilee ham	1 oz	15	3	1	47
chopped ham	1 oz	14	4	2	61
cracked black pepper ham	¾ oz	11	1	tr	24
honey ham	¾ oz	11	1	tr	27
Italian-style cooked ham	¾ oz	9	1	tr	24
Jubilee canned ham	1 oz	13	1	tr	31
Jubilee ham slice	1 oz	13	1	tr	29
Jubilee ham steaks	2 oz	27	2	1	59
smoked cooked ham	2 oz	10	1	tr	23

	Portion	Chol (mg)	Total Fat (g)	Satur'd Fat (g)	Total Calor

❑ POULTRY, FRESH & PROCESSED
See also PROCESSED MEAT & POULTRY PRODUCTS

NOTE: Values are based on the following weights as purchased with giblets & neck:

chicken

broilers or fryers	3.33 lbs
roasting	4.56 lbs
stewing	2.93 lbs
capons	6.5 lbs

duck

domesticated	4.42 lbs
wild	2.26 lbs
goose	8.25 lbs
guinea	1.92 lbs
pheasant	2.15 lbs
quail	0.27 lb
squab	0.67 lb

turkey

all classes	15.47 lbs
fryer-roasters	7.05 lbs
young hens	12.54 lbs
young toms	23.06 lbs

Chicken, Fresh

CHICKEN, BROILERS OR FRYERS

	Portion	Chol (mg)	Total Fat (g)	Satur'd Fat (g)	Total Calor
flesh, skin, giblets, & neck					
fried					
batter-dipped	1 chicken	1,054	180	48	2,987
flour-coated	1 chicken	795	108	29	1,928
roasted	1 chicken	730	90	25	1,598
stewed	1 chicken	726	93	26	1,625
flesh & skin					
fried					
batter-dipped	½ chicken	404	81	22	1,347
flour-coated	½ chicken	283	47	13	844
roasted	½ chicken	263	41	11	715
stewed	½ chicken	262	42	12	730
flesh only					
fried	1 c	131	13	3	307
roasted	1 c	125	10	3	266
stewed	1 c	116	9	3	248

	Portion	Chol (mg)	Total Fat (g)	Satur'd Fat (g)	Total Calor
skin only					
fried					
batter-dipped	½ chicken	140	55	14	748
flour-coated	½ chicken	41	24	7	281
roasted	½ chicken	46	23	6	254
stewed	½ chicken	45	24	7	261
giblets					
fried, flour-coated	1 c	647	20	6	402
simmered	1 c	570	7	2	228
gizzard, simmered	1 c	281	5	2	222
heart, simmered	1 c	350	11	3	268
liver, simmered	1 c	883	8	3	219
light meat w/skin					
fried					
batter-dipped	½ chicken	157	29	8	520
flour-coated	½ chicken	113	16	4	320
roasted	½ chicken	111	14	4	293
stewed	½ chicken	111	15	4	302
dark meat w/skin					
fried					
batter-dipped	½ chicken	247	52	14	828
flour-coated	½ chicken	169	31	8	523
roasted	½ chicken	152	26	7	423
stewed	½ chicken	151	27	7	428
light meat w/out skin					
fried	1 c	125	8	2	268
roasted	1 c	118	6	2	242
stewed	1 c	107	6	2	223
dark meat w/out skin					
fried	1 c	135	16	4	334
roasted	1 c	130	14	4	286
stewed	1 c	123	13	3	269
back, meat & skin					
fried					
batter-dipped	½ back	105	26	7	397
flour-coated	½ back	64	15	4	238
roasted	½ back	46	11	3	159
stewed	½ back	48	11	3	158
back, meat only					
fried	½ back	54	9	2	167
roasted	½ back	36	5	1	96
stewed	½ back	36	5	1	88
breast, meat & skin					
fried					
batter-dipped	½ breast	119	18	5	364
flour-coated	½ breast	88	9	2	218
roasted	½ breast	83	8	2	193
stewed	½ breast	83	8	2	202
breast, meat only					
fried	½ breast	78	4	1	161

	Portion	Chol (mg)	Total Fat (g)	Satur'd Fat (g)	Total Calor
breast, meat only *(cont.)*					
roasted	½ breast	73	3	1	142
stewed	½ breast	73	3	1	144
drumstick, meat & skin					
fried					
batter-dipped	1	62	11	3	193
flour-coated	1	44	7	2	120
roasted	1	48	6	2	112
stewed	1	48	6	2	116
drumstick, meat only					
fried	1	40	3	1	82
roasted	1	41	2	1	76
stewed	1	40	3	1	78
leg (drumstick & thigh), meat & skin					
fried					
batter-dipped	1	142	26	7	431
flour-coated	1	105	16	4	285
roasted	1	105	15	4	265
stewed	1	105	16	4	275
leg (drumstick & thigh), meat only					
fried	1	93	9	2	195
roasted	1	89	8	2	182
stewed	1	90	8	2	187
neck, meat & skin					
fried					
batter-dipped	1	47	12	3	172
flour-coated	1	34	9	2	119
simmered	1	27	7	2	94
neck, meat only					
fried	1	23	3	1	50
simmered	1	14	1	tr	32
thigh, meat & skin					
fried					
batter-dipped	1	80	14	4	238
flour-coated	1	60	9	3	162
roasted	1	58	10	3	153
stewed	1	57	10	3	158
thigh, meat only					
fried	1	53	5	1	113
roasted	1	49	6	2	109
stewed	1	49	5	1	107
wing, meat & skin					
fried					
batter-dipped	1	39	11	3	159
flour-coated	1	26	7	2	103
roasted	1	29	7	2	99
stewed	1	28	7	2	100

	Portion	Chol (mg)	Total Fat (g)	Satur'd Fat (g)	Total Calor
wing, meat only					
fried	1	17	2	1	42
roasted	1	18	2	tr	43
stewed	1	18	2	tr	43
CHICKEN, ROASTING					
flesh & skin, roasted	½ chicken	365	64	18	1,071
flesh only, roasted	1 c	104	9	3	233
giblets, simmered	1 c	517	7	2	239
light meat w/out skin, roasted	1 c	105	6	2	214
dark meat w/out skin, roasted	1 c	104	12	3	250
CHICKEN, STEWING					
flesh, skin, giblets, & neck, stewed	1 chicken	603	107	29	1,636
flesh & skin, stewed	½ chicken	205	49	13	744
flesh only, stewed	1 c	117	17	4	332
giblets, simmered	1 c	515	13	4	281
light meat w/out skin, stewed	1 c	98	11	3	298
dark meat w/out skin, stewed	1 c	132	21	6	361
CHICKEN, CAPONS					
flesh, skin, giblets, & neck, roasted	1 chicken	1,458	165	46	3,211
flesh & skin, roasted	½ chicken	549	74	21	1,457
giblets, simmered	1 c	629	8	3	238

Duck, Fresh

DOMESTICATED

	Portion	Chol (mg)	Total Fat (g)	Satur'd Fat (g)	Total Calor
flesh & skin, roasted	½ duck	320	108	37	1,287
flesh only, roasted	½ duck	198	25	9	445

WILD

	Portion	Chol (mg)	Total Fat (g)	Satur'd Fat (g)	Total Calor
flesh & skin, raw	1 lb of ready-to-cook bird	191	36	12	505
breast, meat only, raw	½ breast	?	4	1	102

Goose, Fresh, Domesticated

	Portion	Chol (mg)	Total Fat (g)	Satur'd Fat (g)	Total Calor
flesh & skin, roasted	½ goose	708	170	53	2,362
flesh only, roasted	½ goose	569	75	27	1,406
liver, raw	1	?	4	1	125

	Portion	Chol (mg)	Total Fat (g)	Satur'd Fat (g)	Total Calor
Guinea, Fresh					
flesh & skin, raw	1 lb of ready-to-cook bird	?	23	?	568
flesh only, raw	1 lb of ready-to-cook bird	?	7	?	304
Pheasant, Fresh					
flesh & skin, raw	1 lb of ready-to-cook bird	?	34	10	670
flesh only, raw	1 lb of ready-to-cook bird	?	12	4	435
breast, meat only, raw	½ breast	?	6	2	243
leg, meat only, raw	1	?	5	2	143
Quail, Fresh					
flesh & skin, raw	1 quail	?	13	4	210
flesh only, raw	1 quail	?	4	1	123
breast, meat only, raw	1	?	2	tr	69
Squab (Pigeon), Fresh					
flesh only, raw	1 squab	?	13	3	239
breast, meat only, raw	1	91	5	1	135
Turkey, Fresh					
TURKEY, ALL CLASSES					
flesh, skin, giblets, & neck, roasted	1 lb of ready-to-cook bird	248	25	7	533
	1 turkey	3,839	380	111	8,245
flesh & skin, roasted	1 lb of ready-to-cook bird	196	23	7	498
	½ turkey	1,514	180	53	3,857
flesh only, roasted	1 c	107	7	2	238
skin only, roasted	½ turkey	281	98	26	1,096
giblets, simmered	1 c	606	7	2	243
gizzard, simmered	1 c	336	6	2	236
heart, simmered	1 c	327	9	3	257
liver, simmered	1 c	876	8	3	237
light meat w/skin, roasted	½ turkey	794	87	25	2,069
dark meat w/skin, roasted	½ turkey	720	93	28	1,789

	Portion	Chol (mg)	Total Fat (g)	Satur'd Fat (g)	Total Calor
light meat w/out skin, roasted	1 c	97	5	1	219
dark meat w/out skin, roasted	1 c	119	10	3	262
back, meat & skin, roasted	½ back	238	38	11	637
breast, meat & skin, roasted	½ breast	643	64	18	1,637
leg, meat & skin, roasted	1	466	54	17	1,133
neck, meat only, simmered	1	186	11	4	274
wing, meat & skin, roasted	1	150	23	6	426
TURKEY, FRYER ROASTERS					
flesh, skin, giblets, & neck, roasted	1 lb of ready-to-cook bird	297	14	4	429
	1 turkey	2,093	100	29	3,029
flesh & skin, roasted	1 lb of ready-to-cook bird	241	13	4	395
	½ turkey	849	46	13	1,392
flesh only, roasted	1 lb of ready-to-cook bird	192	5	2	292
	1 c	138	4	1	210
skin only, roasted	½ turkey	175	28	7	362
light meat w/skin, roasted	½ turkey	413	20	5	711
dark meat w/skin, roasted	½ turkey	436	26	8	680
light meat w/out skin, roasted	1 c	121	2	1	195
dark meat w/out skin, roasted	1 c	157	6	2	227
back					
meat & skin, roasted	½ back	140	11	4	265
meat only, roasted	½ back	91	5	2	164
breast					
meat & skin, roasted	½ breast	310	11	3	526
meat only, roasted	½ breast	255	2	1	413
leg					
meat & skin, roasted	1	171	13	4	418
meat only, roasted	1	267	8	3	355
wing					
meat & skin, roasted	1	104	9	2	186
meat only, roasted	1	61	2	1	98
TURKEY, YOUNG HENS					
flesh, skin, giblets, & neck, roasted	1 lb of ready-to-cook bird	246	28	8	565
	1 turkey	3,092	348	102	7,094
flesh & skin, roasted	½ turkey	1,190	166	48	3,323
flesh only, roasted	1 c	102	8	3	244

	Portion	Chol (mg)	Total Fat (g)	Satur'd Fat (g)	Total Calor
skin only, roasted	½ turkey	207	87	23	945
light meat w/skin, roasted	½ turkey	633	81	23	1,778
dark meat w/skin, roasted	½ turkey	557	85	26	1,544
light meat w/out skin, roasted	1 c	95	5	2	226
dark meat w/out skin, roasted	1 c	111	11	4	268
back, meat & skin, roasted	½ back	185	34	10	551
breast, meat & skin, roasted	½ breast	492	54	15	1,330
leg, meat & skin, roasted	1	365	47	15	955
wing, meat & skin, roasted	1	134	23	6	414

TURKEY, YOUNG TOMS

	Portion	Chol (mg)	Total Fat (g)	Satur'd Fat (g)	Total Calor
flesh, skin, giblets, & neck, roasted	1 lb of ready-to-cook bird	249	23	7	514
	1 turkey	5,745	525	154	11,873
flesh & skin, roasted	1 lb of ready-to-cook bird	197	22	6	482
	½ turkey	2,265	249	73	5,545
flesh only, roasted	1 c	108	7	2	235
skin only, roasted	½ turkey	436	139	36	1,578
light meat w/skin, roasted	½ turkey	1,182	121	34	2,992
dark meat w/skin, roasted	½ turkey	1,081	128	39	2,553
light meat w/out skin, roasted	1 c	97	4	1	215
dark meat w/out skin, roasted	1 c	123	10	3	260
back, meat & skin					
raw	½ back	416	58	16	940
roasted	½ back	358	52	15	903
breast, meat & skin, roasted	½ breast	1,002	98	28	2,510
leg, meat & skin, roasted	1	727	78	24	1,660
wing, meat & skin, roasted	1	192	27	7	524

Poultry, Processed

MECHANICALLY DEBONED POULTRY

	Portion	Chol (mg)	Total Fat (g)	Satur'd Fat (g)	Total Calor
from broiler backs & necks					
w/skin, raw	½ lb	?	56	17	616
w/out skin, raw	½ lb	?	35	11	450
from mature hens, raw	½ lb	324	45	11	551

	Portion	Chol (mg)	Total Fat (g)	Satur'd Fat (g)	Total Calor
from turkey breasts & rib bones, w/ or w/out backs, raw	½ lb	?	36	12	455

TURKEY

	Portion	Chol (mg)	Total Fat (g)	Satur'd Fat (g)	Total Calor
gravy & turkey, frozen	5 oz	?	4	1	95
patties, breaded, battered, fried	2¼ oz	?	12	?	181
	3⅓ oz	?	17	?	266
prebasted turkey					
breast, meat & skin, roasted	½ breast	359	30	8	1,087
thigh, meat & skin, roasted	1	194	27	8	494
roasts, boneless, frozen,	0.43 lb	103	11	?	304
seasoned, light & dark meat, roasted	1.72 lb	413	45	?	1,213
sticks, breaded, battered, fried	2¼ oz	?	11	?	178

▪ BRAND NAME

Armour & Armour Star
broth-basted turkey

	Portion	Chol (mg)	Total Fat (g)	Satur'd Fat (g)	Total Calor
w/sugar	4 oz	?	10	?	180
w/out sugar	4 oz	?	10	?	180
butter-basted turkey	4 oz	?	10	?	190
turkey roast w/gravy					
white meat only	3.69 oz	50	6	?	140
white & dark meat	3.69 oz	50	8	?	150

Land O'Lakes
TURKEY PARTS

	Portion	Chol (mg)	Total Fat (g)	Satur'd Fat (g)	Total Calor
breast	3 oz	50	1	<1	100
drumsticks	3 oz	?	5	2	120
hindquarters roast	3 oz	?	8	3	140
thighs	3 oz	?	10	4	150
wings	3 oz	?	5	2	120

TURKEY PRODUCTS

	Portion	Chol (mg)	Total Fat (g)	Satur'd Fat (g)	Total Calor
breast fillets w/cheese	5 oz	35	16	5	300
patties	2¼ oz	30	11	3	170
sticks	2 oz	25	10	3	150

WHOLE TURKEY

	Portion	Chol (mg)	Total Fat (g)	Satur'd Fat (g)	Total Calor
butter-basted young turkey	3 oz	85	8	3	140
self-basting (broth) young turkey	3 oz	77	5	2	120
young turkey	3 oz	65	7	2	130

	Portion	Chol (mg)	Total Fat (g)	Satur'd Fat (g)	Total Calor
Tyson					
FULLY COOKED CHICKEN					
Batter Gold	about 3½ oz	85	19	2	285
buttermilk	about 3½ oz	71	20	1	285
Delecta Delicious	about 3½ oz	82	19	2	305
Heat N Serve (oven ready)	about 3½ oz	74	17	tr	270
Honey Stung	about 3½ oz	90	14	1	260
lightly breaded	about 3½ oz	94	14	1	255
POULTRY PRODUCTS					
breast patties	3 oz	?	17	?	240
breast strips	about 3½ oz	43	13	1	270
chicken pattie	about 3½ oz	58	19	3	275
Chick'n Cheddar	3 oz	?	17	?	260
Chick'n Chunks	3 oz = 6 pieces	?	16	?	250
Chick'n Dippers	3 oz = 4 dippers	?	16	?	250
Chick'n Sticks	3 oz = 3 pieces	?	15	?	240
Heat N Serve	about 3½ oz	53	19	1	280
Sandwich Mate	about 3½ oz	40	20	2	315
School Lunch pattie	about 3½ oz	33	20	2	290
Southern Fried Chunks	3 oz	?	16	?	250
Swiss 'n Bacon	3 oz	?	20	?	280
turkey patties	3 oz	?	14	?	220
READY-TO-COOK POULTRY					
boneless breast	about 3½ oz	50	13	1	205
Cornish & split Cornish	about 3½ oz	52	14	1	240
IQF chicken & split broilers	about 3½ oz	58	15	1	245
prebreaded marinated chicken	about 3½ oz	65	17	1	285

	Portion	Chol (mg)	Total Fat (g)	Satur'd Fat (g)	Total Calor

❏ **POULTRY SPREADS** *See* PROCESSED MEAT & POULTRY PRODUCTS

❏ **PRESERVES** *See* FRUIT SPREADS

❏ **PROCESSED MEAT & POULTRY PRODUCTS: SAUSAGES, FRANKFURTERS, COLD CUTS, PÂTÉS, & SPREADS**
See also BEEF, FRESH & CURED; PORK, FRESH & CURED; POULTRY, FRESH & PROCESSED

	Portion	Chol (mg)	Total Fat (g)	Satur'd Fat (g)	Total Calor
bacon & Canadian-style bacon *See* PORK, FRESH & CURED					
barbecue loaf, pork, beef	1 oz	11	3	1	49
beef sausage, smoked	1 oz	19	8	3	89
	1½ oz	29	12	5	134
beerwurst, beer salami					
beef	0.2 oz	3	2	1	19
	0.8 oz	13	7	3	75
pork	0.2 oz	4	1	tr	14
	0.8 oz	13	4	1	55
berliner, pork, beef	1 oz	13	5	2	65
blood sausage	1 oz	34	10	4	107
bockwurst, raw (pork, veal)	2½ oz	?	18	7	200
	1 oz	?	8	3	87
bologna					
beef	0.8 oz	13	7	3	72
	1 oz	16	8	3	89
beef & pork	0.8 oz	13	7	2	73
	1 oz	16	8	3	89
pork	0.8 oz	14	5	2	57
	1 oz	17	6	2	70
turkey	1 oz	28	4	?	57
bratwurst, cooked, pork	3 oz	51	22	8	256
	1 oz	17	7	3	85
braunschweiger (a liver sausage), pork	0.6 oz	28	6	2	65
	1 oz	44	9	3	102
breakfast strips *See* BEEF, FRESH & CURED; PORK, FRESH & CURED					
brotwurst, pork, beef	2½ oz	44	19	7	226
	1 oz	18	8	3	92
cheesefurter, pork, beef	1½ oz	29	12	5	141
chicken, canned, boned, w/broth	5 oz	?	11	3	234
chicken roll, light meat	2 oz	28	4	1	90
	6 oz	85	13	3	271

	Portion	Chol (mg)	Total Fat (g)	Satur'd Fat (g)	Total Calor
chicken spread, canned	1 T	?	2	?	25
	1 oz	?	3	?	55
chorizo, pork & beef	1 oz	?	11	4	?
corned beef, braised *See* BEEF, FRESH & CURED					
corned beef, canned	1 oz	24	4	2	71
corned beef loaf, jellied	1 oz	12	2	1	46
dried beef	1 oz	?	1	tr	47
Dutch brand loaf, pork, beef	1 oz	13	5	2	68
frankfurter					
beef	2 oz	27	17	7	184
	1.6 oz	22	13	5	145
beef & pork	2 oz	29	17	6	183
	1.6 oz	22	13	5	144
chicken	1.6 oz	45	9	2	116
	1 oz	28	6	2	73
turkey	1.6 oz	48	8	?	102
	1 oz	30	5	?	64
ham, boneless or canned *See* PORK, FRESH & CURED					
ham, chopped	1 oz	15	5	2	65
ham, chopped, canned	1 oz	14	5	2	68
ham, minced	1 oz	20	6	2	75
ham & cheese loaf or roll	1 oz	16	6	2	73
ham & cheese spread	1 T	9	3	1	37
	1 oz	17	5	2	69
ham salad spread	1 T	6	2	1	32
	1 oz	10	4	1	61
head cheese, pork	1 oz	23	4	1	60
honey loaf, pork, beef	1 oz	10	1	tr	36
honey roll sausage, beef	1 oz	14	3	1	52
hot dog *See* frankfurter, *above*					
Italian sausage, pork					
raw	3.2 oz	69	29	10	315
	4 oz	86	35	13	391
cooked	2.3 oz	52	17	6	216
	2.9 oz	65	21	8	268
kielbasa, pork, beef	1 oz	19	8	3	88
knockwurst, pork, beef	2.4 oz	39	19	7	209
	1 oz	16	8	3	87
Lebanon bologna, beef	0.8 oz	15	3	1	52
	1 oz	19	4	2	64
liver cheese, pork	1.3 oz	66	10	3	115
	1 oz	49	7	3	86
liver sausage (liverwurst), pork	1 oz	45	8	3	93
luncheon meat					
beef, jellied	1 oz	?	1	tr	31
beef, loaved	1 oz	18	7	3	87
beef, thin-sliced	1 oz	12	1	tr	35
pork, beef	1 oz	15	9	3	100
pork, canned	1 oz	18	9	3	95

	Portion	Chol (mg)	Total Fat (g)	Satur'd Fat (g)	Total Calor
luncheon sausage, pork &	0.8 oz	15	5	2	60
beef	1 oz	18	6	2	74
mortadella, beef, pork	about ½ oz	8	4	1	47
	1 oz	16	7	3	88
olive loaf, pork	1 oz	11	5	2	67
pastrami					
beef	1 oz	26	8	3	99
turkey	2 oz	?	4	1	80
	8 oz	?	14	4	320
pâté					
chicken liver, canned	1 T	?	2	?	26
	1 oz	?	4	?	57
goose liver, smoked,	1 T	20	6	?	60
canned	1 oz	43	12	?	131
liver (not specified),	1 T	?	4	?	41
canned	1 oz	?	8	?	90
peppered loaf, pork, beef	1 oz	13	2	1	42
pepperoni, pork, beef	8.8 oz	?	110	40	1,248
	0.2 oz	?	2	1	27
pickle & pimento loaf, pork	1 oz	10	6	2	74
picnic loaf, pork, beef	1 oz	11	5	2	66
Polish sausage, pork	8 oz	158	65	23	739
	1 oz	20	8	3	92
pork & beef sausage,	about 1 oz	?	10	4	107
fresh, cooked	about ½ oz	?	5	2	52
pork sausage, country	about 1 oz	22	8	3	100
style, fresh, cooked	about ½ oz	11	4	1	48
salami					
cooked					
beef	0.8 oz	14	5	2	58
	1 oz	17	6	2	72
beef & pork	0.8 oz	15	5	2	57
	1 oz	18	6	2	71
turkey	2 oz	46	8	?	111
	8 oz	186	31	?	446
dry or hard					
pork	0.35 oz	?	3	1	41
	4 oz	?	38	13	460
pork, beef	0.35 oz	8	3	1	42
	4 oz	89	39	14	472
sandwich spread					
pork, beef	1 T	6	3	1	35
	1 oz	11	5	2	67
poultry salad	1 T	4	2	tr	26
	1 oz	9	4	1	57
smoked chopped beef	1 oz	13	1	1	38
smoked link sausage					
pork, grilled	2.4 oz	46	22	8	265
	about ½ oz	11	5	2	62
pork & beef	2.4 oz	48	21	7	229
	about ½ oz	11	5	2	54

	Portion	Chol (mg)	Total Fat (g)	Satur'd Fat (g)	Total Calor
smoked link sausage *(cont.)*					
flour & nonfat dry milk	2.4 oz	59	15	5	182
added	about ½ oz	14	3	1	43
nonfat dry milk added	2.4 oz	44	19	7	213
	about ½ oz	10	4	2	50
Thuringer, cervelat, sum-	0.8 oz	16	7	3	80
mer sausage: beef, pork	1 oz	19	8	3	98
turkey					
canned, boned, w/broth	5 oz	?	10	3	231
diced, light & dark, sea-	1 oz	?	2	1	39
soned	½ lb	?	14	4	313
turkey breast meat	0.7 oz	9	tr	tr	23
turkey ham (cured turkey	2 oz	?	3	1	73
thigh meat)	8 oz	?	12	4	291
turkey loaf, breast meat	1½ oz	17	1	tr	47
	6 oz	69	3	1	187
turkey pastrami *See* pastrami: turkey, *above*					
turkey roll, light meat	1 oz	12	2	1	42
turkey roll, light & dark meat	1 oz	16	2	1	42
Vienna sausage, canned, beef & pork	0.6 oz	8	4	1	45

▪ BRAND NAME

Armour & Armour Star
FRANKFURTERS

	Portion	Chol (mg)	Total Fat (g)	Satur'd Fat (g)	Total Calor
beef	1.6 oz	20	13	?	150
lower salt Jumbo & Jumbo Beef	2 oz	30	15	?	170
regular Jumbo & Jumbo Beef	2 oz	30	18	?	190
Giant All Meat	1.6 oz	25	13	?	150
Giant Beef	1 link	25	17	?	180
Giant Great 8 Beef	2 oz	25	17	?	180
Giant Great 8 Meat	2 oz	28	17	?	180
turkey	2 oz	50	8	?	110

LUNCHEON MEATS

	Portion	Chol (mg)	Total Fat (g)	Satur'd Fat (g)	Total Calor
barbecue loaf	1 oz	10	3	?	50
bologna or beef bologna	1 oz	15	9	?	100
lower salt	1 oz	15	8	?	90
liverwurst	1 oz	45	8	?	90
Old Fashioned Loaf	1 oz	15	7	?	80
pepperoni					
Italian	1 oz	20	11	?	130
sliced	1 oz	20	11	?	130

	Portion	Chol (mg)	Total Fat (g)	Satur'd Fat (g)	Total Calor
salami					
Genoa, sliced	1 oz	30	10	?	110
hard	1 oz	20	10	?	120
Italian, hard	1 oz	20	10	?	120
lower salt	1 oz	20	7	?	80
sliced	1 oz	20	10	?	120
spiced luncheon meat					
regular	3 oz	?	25	?	280
w/chicken	3 oz	70	24	?	280
summer sausage, cheese	1 oz	20	8	?	100
turkey bologna	4 oz	95	16	?	220
turkey cotto salami	4 oz	70	11	?	180
turkey ham	4 oz	60	4	?	140
turkey meat loaf	3 oz	50	8	?	160
turkey pastrami	4 oz	65	5	?	140
turkey roll, Magic Slice, cooked, white or white & dark	3 oz	50	5	?	120

MEAT PRODUCTS, CANNED

	Portion	Chol (mg)	Total Fat (g)	Satur'd Fat (g)	Total Calor
corned beef hash	1½ oz	?	27	?	390
deviled ham	1½ oz	?	9	?	110
Deviled Treet	1½ oz	?	10	?	120
potted meat	1½ oz	?	6	?	80
roast beef hash	7½ oz	?	21	?	350
sliced dried beef	1 oz	?	2	?	60
sloppy joes, beef	about 7½ oz	?	25	?	390
smoked Vienna sausage	2 oz	?	17	?	180
Vienna sausage in beef stock	2 oz	?	17	?	180

SAUSAGES

	Portion	Chol (mg)	Total Fat (g)	Satur'd Fat (g)	Total Calor
sausage links, regular or lower salt, uncooked	1 oz	?	11	?	110
sausage patties, regular or lower salt, uncooked	1½ oz	?	16	?	160
sausage rolls, regular or lower salt, uncooked	1 oz	?	11	?	110

Carl Buddig Luncheon Meats

	Portion	Chol (mg)	Total Fat (g)	Satur'd Fat (g)	Total Calor
beef	1 oz	16	2	1	40
chicken	1 oz	12	3	1	50
corned beef	1 oz	16	2	1	40
ham	1 oz	20	3	1	50
pastrami	1 oz	16	2	1	40
turkey	1 oz	6	3	1	50
turkey ham	1 oz	19	2	1	40
turkey salami	1 oz	19	2	1	40

Health Valley

	Portion	Chol (mg)	Total Fat (g)	Satur'd Fat (g)	Total Calor
bologna					
beef, sliced	3½ oz	?	30	?	310

	Portion	Chol (mg)	Total Fat (g)	Satur'd Fat (g)	Total Calor
bologna *(cont.)*					
chicken	3½ oz	?	30	?	300
frankfurters					
beef	3½ oz	?	25	?	288
chicken	3½ oz	?	26	?	290
turkey	3½ oz	?	20	?	238
knockwurst	3½ oz	?	25	?	280
pork, sliced, breakfast	3½ oz	?	60	?	560
salami, sliced	3½ oz	?	35	?	400
Land O'Lakes					
diced turkey, white & dark mixed	3 oz	35	6	2	120
turkey ham	3 oz	55	2	<1	100
Louis Rich					
barbecued breast of turkey	1 oz	10	1	tr	38
hickory smoked breast of turkey	1 oz	13	1	tr	35
oven roasted breast of turkey	1 oz	10	1	tr	36
oven roasted chicken breast	1 oz	14	2	1	39
smoked turkey breast, sliced	¾ oz	7	tr	tr	21
turkey franks	1 link = 1.58 oz	40	9	3	103
turkey ham	1 oz	18	1	1	34
turkey pastrami	1 oz	17	1	tr	33
turkey salami	1 oz	19	4	1	52
turkey smoked sausage	1 oz	19	4	1	55
Oscar Mayer					
FRANKFURTERS					
beef	1 link	27	13	6	144
cheese	1 link	30	13	5	145
little wieners	1 link	5	3	1	28
wieners	1 link	27	13	5	144
LUNCHEON MEATS					
Bar-B-Q loaf	1 oz	13	3	1	47
beef bologna	1 oz	16	8	4	90
beef cotto salami	0.8 oz	15	3	2	45
beef salami for beer	0.8 oz	21	6	3	67
beef summer sausage	0.8 oz	17	6	3	73
bologna	1 oz	17	8	3	90
braunschweiger liver sausage	1 oz	41	9	3	96
corned beef	0.6 oz	5	tr	tr	16
cotto salami	0.8 oz	15	4	2	54
Genoa salami	0.3 oz	8	3	1	35
German brand braunschweiger	1 oz	46	8	3	94

	Portion	Chol (mg)	Total Fat (g)	Satur'd Fat (g)	Total Calor
ham *See* PORK, FRESH & CURED					
ham & cheese loaf	1 oz	17	6	2	76
hard salami	0.3 oz	7	3	1	34
head cheese	1 oz	21	4	1	55
honey loaf	1 oz	12	1	tr	35
Italian-style beef	0.6 oz	6	1	tr	18
liver cheese	1.3 oz	75	10	4	116
luncheon meat	1 oz	16	9	4	99
Luxury Loaf	1 oz	13	1	1	38
New England brand sausage	0.8 oz	13	2	1	31
Old Fashioned Loaf	1 oz	14	4	2	64
olive loaf	1 oz	10	4	2	63
pastrami	0.6 oz	5	tr	tr	17
peppered loaf	1 oz	13	2	1	43
pickle & pimiento loaf	1 oz	10	4	2	64
picnic loaf	1 oz	12	4	2	62
summer sausage	0.8 oz	17	7	3	73
SAUSAGES					
Beef Smokies	1 link	27	11	5	122
Little Friers, pork	1 link	16	7	3	77
Little Smokies	1 link	6	3	1	28
Smokie Links	1 link	27	11	4	124
SLICED CHICKEN & TURKEY					
smoked chicken breast	1 oz	11	1	tr	27
smoked turkey breast	0.7 oz	7	tr	tr	20
SPREADS					
braunschweiger liver sausage	1 oz	50	9	3	95
ham & cheese	1 oz	16	5	2	66
ham salad	1 oz	11	4	2	62
sandwich	1 oz	10	5	2	67
Swanson					
chunk premium white chicken, canned	2½ oz	?	2	?	90
chunk-style Mixin' Chicken, canned	2½ oz	?	8	?	130
chunk white & dark chicken, canned	2½ oz	?	4	?	100
chunky chicken spread	1 oz	?	4	?	60
Tyson					
all white cooked chicken fryer meat	about 3½ oz	40	3	1	166
breast of chicken roll, whole & diced	about 3½ oz	47	9	2	155

	Portion	Chol (mg)	Total Fat (g)	Satur'd Fat (g)	Total Calor
chicken bologna	about 3½ oz	60	18	1	230
chicken corn dogs	about 3½ oz	55	14	1	280
chicken franks	about 3½ oz	68	25	2	285
Liberty Roll, whole & diced	about 3½ oz	53	12	3	185
natural proportioned cooked chicken meat	about 3½ oz	53	5	1	170

❏ **PUDDING DESSERTS, FROZEN**
See DESSERTS, FROZEN

❏ **PUDDINGS & PIE FILLINGS**
See DESSERTS: CUSTARDS, GELATINS,
PUDDINGS, & PIE FILLINGS

❏ **RELISHES** *See* PICKLES, OLIVES,
RELISHES, & CHUTNEYS

❏ **RICE & GRAINS, PLAIN & PREPARED**
See also VEGETABLES, PLAIN & PREPARED

barley, pearled, light, un-cooked	1 c	0	2	tr	700
bulgur, uncooked	1 c	0	3	1	600
hominy grits *See* corn grits, *under* BREAKFAST CEREALS, COLD & HOT					
popcorn *See* SNACKS					
rice					
brown, cooked, hot	1 c	0	1	tr	230
white, enriched					
raw	1 c	0	1	tr	670
cooked, hot	1 c	6	tr	tr	225
instant, ready-to-serve, hot	1 c	0	0	tr	180
parboiled, raw	1 c	0	1	tr	685
parboiled, cooked, hot	1 c	0	tr	tr	185

	Portion	Chol (mg)	Total Fat (g)	Satur'd Fat (g)	Total Calor

- **BRAND NAME**

Arrowhead Mills
PLAIN RICE & GRAINS

barley, pearled, or barley flakes	2 oz	0	1	?	200
buckwheat groats, brown or white	2 oz	0	1	?	190
bulgur wheat	2 oz	0	1	?	200
corn					
blue	2 oz	0	3	?	210
yellow	2 oz	0	2	?	210
millet	2 oz	0	1	?	90
oat flakes	2 oz	0	4	?	220
oat groats	2 oz	0	4	?	220
quinoa	2 oz	0	3	?	200
rice, brown: long, long basmati, medium, or short	2 oz	0	1	?	200
rye or rye flakes	2 oz	0	1	?	190
triticale or triticale flakes	2 oz	0	1	?	190
wheat, hard, red, winter, or soft pastry	2 oz	0	1	?	190
wheat flakes	2 oz	0	1	?	210

PREPARED RICE & GRAINS

quick brown rice					
regular	2 oz	0	1	?	200
Spanish style	¼ of 5.65 oz pkg	0	1	?	150
vegetable herb	¼ of 5.6 oz pkg	0	1	?	150
wild rice & herbs	¼ of 5.35 oz pkg	0	1	?	140

Birds Eye International Rice Recipes

French style	3.3 oz	0	0	0	110
Italian style	3.3 oz	0	1	?	120
Spanish style	3.3 oz	0	0	0	110

Carolina Rice

extra long grain, enriched	about ½ c cooked	0	0	0	100
long grain, enriched, pre-cooked instant	about ½ c cooked	0	0	0	110

Chun King

rice mix	¼ oz	0	0	0	20

Fearn

Naturfresh corn germ	¼ c or 1 oz	0	7	1	130
Naturfresh raw wheat germ	¼ c or 1 oz	0	3	tr	100

	Portion	Chol (mg)	Total Fat (g)	Satur'd Fat (g)	Total Calor
Featherweight					
Spanish rice	7½ oz	?	0	?	140
Health Valley					
amaranth pilaf, regular or low-salt	4 oz	0	3	?	90
Mahatma					
long grain rice, enriched	about ½ c cooked	0	0	0	100
long grain rice, enriched, precooked instant	about ½ c cooked	0	0	0	110
natural long grain rice, brown	about ½ c cooked	0	0	0	110
Minute Rice					
drumstick mix, w/salted butter	½ c	10	4	?	150
fried rice mix, w/oil	½ c	0	5	?	160
long grain & wild rice mix, w/salted butter	½ c	10	4	?	150
rib roast mix, w/salted butter	½ c	10	4	?	150
rice, w/out salt or butter	⅔ c	0	0	0	120
Quaker Oats					
Scotch brand medium pearled barley	¼ c	?	1	?	172
Scotch brand quick pearled barley	¼ c	?	1	?	172
Rice-A-Roni					
MICROWAVE LONG GRAIN & WILD RICE MIXES					
original flavor w/herbs & seasoning, prepared	½ c	?	4	?	140
chicken flavor & mushroom, prepared	½ c	?	4	?	140
RICE & PASTA MIXES					
beef flavor, prepared	½ c	?	5	?	170
beef flavor & mushroom, prepared	½ c	?	4	?	150
chicken & mushroom flavor, prepared	½ c	?	7	?	180
chicken flavor, prepared	½ c	?	5	?	170
chicken flavor/chicken broth w/herbs, twin pack, prepared	⅔ c	?	7	?	220
chicken flavor & vegetables, prepared	½ c	?	4	?	140
fried rice w/almonds, prepared	½ c	?	5	?	140
herbs & butter, prepared	½ c	?	4	?	130
rice pilaf, prepared	½ c	?	6	?	190

	Portion	Chol (mg)	Total Fat (g)	Satur'd Fat (g)	Total Calor
risotto, prepared	¾ c	?	7	?	210
Spanish rice, prepared	½ c	?	4	?	140
Stroganoff w/sour cream sauce, prepared	½ c	?	8	?	200
RICE MIXES					
brown & wild rice w/ mushrooms, prepared	½ c	?	8	?	180
long grain & wild rice w/ herbs & seasoning, prepared	½ c	?	5	?	140
yellow rice dinner, prepared	¾ c	?	7	?	250
River					
enriched rice	about ½ c cooked	0	0	0	100
natural long grain rice, brown	about ½ c cooked	0	0	0	110
Riviana Make-It-Easy					
beef-flavored rice & vermicelli mix	⅙ of 8 oz box or about ½ c cooked	?	1	?	130
chicken-flavored rice & vermicelli mix	⅙ of 8 oz box or about ½ c cooked	?	1	?	130
Stouffer					
apple pecan rice	½ of 5⅞ oz pkg	?	4	?	130
Rice Medley	3 oz	?	2	?	110
Success					
enriched, precooked, natural long grain rice	about ½ c cooked	0	0	0	100
Van Camp's					
Golden Hominy	1 c	0	1	?	128
Spanish rice	1 c	?	3	?	150
Water Maid					
enriched rice	about ½ c cooked	0	0	0	100

❑ **ROLLS** *See* BREADS, ROLLS, BISCUITS, & MUFFINS

	Portion	Chol (mg)	Total Fat (g)	Satur'd Fat (g)	Total Calor

❑ SALAD DRESSINGS, MAYONNAISE, VINEGAR, & DIPS

Mayonnaise, Commercial

	Portion	Chol (mg)	Total Fat (g)	Satur'd Fat (g)	Total Calor
mayonnaise					
safflower & soybean	1 c	?	175	19	1,577
	1 T	?	11	1	99
soybean	1 c	130	175	26	1,577
	1 T	8	11	2	99
mayonnaise, imitation					
milk, cream	1 c	103	12	7	232
	1 T	6	1	tr	15
soybean	1 c	58	46	8	556
	1 T	4	3	1	35
soybean w/out cholesterol	1 c	0	107	17	1,084
	1 T	0	7	1	68
mayonnaise-type dressing					
regular	1 c	60	78	12	916
	1 T	4	5	1	57
low-cal	1 T	?	2	?	19

Salad Dressings

	Portion	Chol (mg)	Total Fat (g)	Satur'd Fat (g)	Total Calor
bleu cheese, commercial					
regular	1 c	?	128	24	1,235
	1 T	?	8	2	77
low-cal	1 T	?	1	?	11
Caesar, commercial	1 T	?	7	?	70
cole slaw, commercial low-cal	1 T	?	3	?	31
cooked, homemade	1 c	?	24	7	400
	1 T	?	2	1	25
French commercial					
regular	1 c	?	102	24	1,074
	1 T	?	6	2	67
creamy	1 T	?	7	?	70
low-cal	1 c	15	15	2	349
	1 T	1	1	tr	22
homemade	1 c	?	154	28	1,388
	1 T	?	10	2	88
Green Goddess, commercial					
regular	1 T	?	7	?	68
low-cal	1 T	?	2	?	27
Italian, commercial					
regular	1 c	?	114	16	1,098
	1 T	?	7	1	69
creamy	1 T	?	5	?	52

	Portion	Chol (mg)	Total Fat (g)	Satur'd Fat (g)	Total Calor
low-cal	1 c	14	24	3	253
	1 T	1	2	tr	16
Russian, commercial					
regular	1 c	?	125	18	1,210
	1 T	?	8	1	76
low-cal	1 c	15	10	2	368
	1 T	1	1	tr	23
poppy seed	1 oz	?	11	?	121
sesame seed, commercial	1 c	0	111	15	1,086
	1 T	0	7	1	68
sweet & sour, commercial	1 T	?	tr	?	29
Thousand Island, commercial					
regular	1 c	?	89	15	943
	1 T	?	6	1	59
low-cal	1 c	38	26	4	389
	1 T	2	2	tr	24
vinegar & oil, homemade	1 c	?	125	23	1,122
	1 T	?	8	2	72
vinegar (red wine) & oil, commercial	1 oz	?	9	?	103

Vinegar

cider	1 T	0	0	0	tr
distilled	1 T	0	0	0	2

■ BRAND NAME

Featherweight
LOW-SALT DRESSINGS

Soyamaise	1 T	?	11	?	100

LOW-SALT, LOW-CAL DRESSINGS

Caesar	1 T	?	1	?	14
creamy cucumber	1 T	?	0	0	4
French	1 T	?	0	0	14
herb	1 T	?	0	0	6
Italian	1 T	?	0	0	4
New Bleu	1 T	?	0	0	4
red wine vinegar	1 T	?	0	0	6
Russian	1 T	?	0	0	6
Thousand Island	1 T	?	0	0	18
Zesty Tomato	1 T	?	0	0	2

Good Seasons Salad Dressing Mixes

bleu cheese & herbs, w/ vinegar, water, & salad oil	1 T	0	9	?	80

	Portion	Chol (mg)	Total Fat (g)	Satur'd Fat (g)	Total Calor
Buttermilk Farm Style, w/ whole milk & mayonnaise	1 T	5	6	?	60
cheese garlic, w/vinegar, water, & salad oil	1 T	0	9	?	80
cheese Italian, w/vinegar, water, & salad oil	1 T	0	9	?	80
classic herb, w/vinegar, water, & salad oil	1 T	0	9	?	80
garlic & herbs, w/vinegar, water, & salad oil	1 T	0	9	?	80
Italian, w/vinegar, water, & salad oil	1 T	0	9	?	80
lemon & herbs, w/vinegar, water, & salad oil	1 T	0	9	?	80
lite Italian, w/vinegar, water, & salad oil	1 T	0	3	?	25
no-oil Italian, w/vinegar & water	1 T	0	0	0	6
Hellman's					
Real mayonnaise	1 T	5	11	2	100
sandwich spread	1 T	5	5	1	50
tartar sauce	1 T	5	8	1	70
Land O'Lakes					
dips, flavored, dairy	2 oz	10	5	3	70
Life All Natural					
avocado dressing/dip w/ tofu	½ oz	0	7	?	70
creamy salad dressing, egg-free, low-cholesterol	½ oz	0	4	?	39
garlic dressing/dip w/tofu	½ oz	0	7	?	70
mayonnaise-style dressing, egg-free, low-cholesterol	½ oz	0	8	?	71
tofu dressing/dip	½ oz	0	7	?	75
Ortega					
Acapulco Dip	1 oz	0	0	0	8
Regina					
wine vinegars, all flavors	1 fl oz	?	0	?	4

❑ **SALADS, COMMERCIALLY PREPARED**
See FAST FOODS; FRUIT, FRESH
& PROCESSED; VEGETABLES, PLAIN &
PREPARED

	Portion	Chol (mg)	Total Fat (g)	Satur'd Fat (g)	Total Calor

◻ SAUCES, DESSERT *See* DESSERT SAUCES, SYRUPS, & TOPPINGS

◻ SAUCES, GRAVIES, & CONDIMENTS
See also FRUIT, FRESH & PROCESSED; PICKLES, OLIVES, RELISHES, & CHUTNEYS

Condiments

	Portion	Chol (mg)	Total Fat (g)	Satur'd Fat (g)	Total Calor
catsup	1 c	0	1	tr	290
mustard, prepared, yellow	1 t	0	tr	tr	5

Gravies

	Portion	Chol (mg)	Total Fat (g)	Satur'd Fat (g)	Total Calor
au jus					
canned	1 c	1	tr	tr	38
	10½ oz	1	1	tr	48
dehydrated, prepared w/ water	1 c	1	1	tr	19
	21.7 oz	2	2	1	48
beef, canned	1 c	7	5	3	124
	10¼ oz	9	7	3	155
brown, dehydrated, prepared w/water	1 c	tr	tr	tr	9
	9.7 oz	tr	tr	tr	9
chicken					
canned	1 c	5	14	3	189
	10½ oz	6	17	4	236
dehydrated, prepared w/ water	1 c	3	2	1	83
mushroom					
canned	1 c	0	6	1	120
	10½ oz	0	8	1	150
dehydrated, prepared w/ water	1 c	1	1	1	70
onion, dehydrated, prepared w/water	1 c	1	1	tr	80
pork, dehydrated, prepared w/water	1 c	3	2	1	76
turkey					
canned	1 c	5	5	1	122
	10½ oz	6	6	2	152
dehydrated, prepared w/ water	1 c	3	2	1	87

	Portion	Chol (mg)	Total Fat (g)	Satur'd Fat (g)	Total Calor
Sauces					
barbecue, ready-to-serve	1 c	0	5	1	188
béarnaise					
dehydrated	0.9 oz	tr	2	tr	90
dehydrated, prepared w/	1 c	189	68	42	701
milk & butter	13½ oz	283	102	63	1,052
cheese					
dehydrated	1.2 oz	18	9	4	158
dehydrated, prepared w/ whole milk	1 c	53	17	9	307
curry					
dehydrated	1.2 oz	tr	8	1	151
dehydrated, prepared w/	1 c	35	15	6	270
whole milk	12 oz	44	18	8	337
hollandaise, dehydrated					
w/butterfat	1.2 oz	40	16	9	187
w/butterfat, prepared w/	1 c	51	20	12	237
water	7.2 oz	40	16	9	187
w/vegetable oil	1 oz	tr	2	tr	93
w/vegetable oil, prepared	1 c	189	68	42	703
w/milk & butter	13½ oz	283	102	63	1,055
marinara, canned	1 c	0	8	1	171
	15½ oz	0	15	2	300
mushroom					
dehydrated	1 oz	0	3	tr	99
dehydrated, prepared w/	1 c	34	10	5	228
whole milk	11.7 oz	43	13	7	285
sour cream					
dehydrated	1.2 oz	28	11	6	180
dehydrated, prepared w/	1 c	91	30	16	509
whole milk	5½ oz	46	15	8	255
soy *See* SOYBEANS & SOYBEAN PRODUCTS					
spaghetti					
canned	1 c	0	12	2	272
	15½ oz	0	21	3	479
dehydrated	0.35 oz	0	tr	tr	28
	1½ oz	0	tr	tr	118
dehydrated, w/mush-	0.35 oz	3	1	1	30
rooms	1.4 oz	11	4	2	118
Stroganoff					
dehydrated	1.6 oz	12	4	3	161
dehydrated, prepared w/	1 c	38	11	7	271
whole milk & water	11.2 oz	41	12	7	292
sweet & sour					
dehydrated	2 oz	0	tr	tr	220
dehydrated, prepared w/	1 c	0	tr	tr	294
water & vinegar	8.3 oz	0	tr	tr	220
tamari *See* SOYBEANS & SOYBEAN PRODUCTS					

	Portion	Chol (mg)	Total Fat (g)	Satur'd Fat (g)	Total Calor
teriyaki *See* SOYBEANS & SOYBEAN PRODUCTS					
tomato, canned	½ c	0	tr	tr	37
Spanish style	½ c	0	tr	tr	40
w/herbs & cheese	½ c	?	2	1	72
w/mushrooms	½ c	0	tr	tr	42
w/onions	½ c	0	tr	tr	52
w/onions, green peppers, & celery	½ c	0	1	tr	50
w/tomato tidbits	½ c	0	tr	tr	39
tomato paste & puree *See* VEGETABLES, PLAIN & PREPARED					
white					
dehydrated	1.7 oz	tr	13	3	230
dehydrated, prepared w/ whole milk	1 c	34	13	6	241
	23.2 oz	86	34	16	602

▪ BRAND NAME

A-1
steak sauce	1 T	?	0	?	12

Chun King
mustard, brown	1 t	?	0	?	4
sauce/glaze mix for sweet & sour entree	3.8 oz	0	0	0	370
sweet & sour sauce	1.8 oz	?	0	?	60

Escoffier
Sauce Diable	1 T	?	0	?	20
Sauce Robert	1 T	?	0	?	20

Franco-American Gravies
au jus	2 oz	?	0	?	5
beef	2 oz	?	1	?	25
brown, w/onions	2 oz	?	1	?	25
chicken	2 oz	?	4	?	50
chicken giblet	2 oz	?	2	?	30
mushroom	2 oz	?	1	?	25
pork	2 oz	?	3	?	40
turkey	2 oz	?	2	?	30

Fresh Chef Sauces
Bolognese	4 oz	?	7	?	130
pesto	4 oz	?	60	?	630
red clam	4 oz	?	4	?	90
tomato	4 oz	?	11	?	160
white clam	4 oz	?	10	?	130

Grey Poupon
Dijon mustard	1 T	?	1	?	18

Health Valley
Catch-Up, regular or no salt	1 T	0	tr	?	16

	Portion	Chol (mg)	Total Fat (g)	Satur'd Fat (g)	Total Calor
tomato sauce, regular or no salt	4 oz	0	0	?	30
Life All Natural					
English mustard	¼ oz	?	1	?	11
horseradish sauce	¼ fl oz	?	tr	?	7
steak sauce	½ oz	0	tr	?	11
tartar sauce, egg-free, low-cholesterol	¼ fl oz	0	2	?	19
tomato catsup	½ oz	0	0	0	11
Worcestershire sauce	¼ oz	0	tr	?	5
Open Pit					
all barbecue sauces	1 T	0	0	0	25
Ortega					
enchilada sauce, mild or hot	1 oz	?	0	?	12
green chile salsa					
mild or medium	1 oz	?	0	?	8
hot	1 oz	?	0	?	10
Picante salsa	1 oz	?	0	?	10
Ranchera salsa	1 oz	?	0	?	12
taco salsa, mild or hot	1 oz	?	0	?	10
taco sauce, mild or hot	1 oz	?	0	?	12
Western-style taco sauce	1 oz	?	0	?	8
Prego					
Al Fresco Garden tomato sauce	4 oz	?	5	?	100
Prego Plus					
w/beef sirloin & onion	4 oz	?	7	?	160
w/mushrooms & chunk	4 oz	?	5	?	130
w/sausage & green peppers	4 oz	?	9	?	170
w/veal & sliced mushrooms	4 oz	?	5	?	150
spaghetti sauce	4 oz	?	6	?	140
spaghetti sauce, meat-flavored	4 oz	?	6	?	150
Steak Supreme					
steak sauce	1 T	?	0	?	20
Tabasco					
Tabasco sauce	¼ t	0	tr	tr	1
Wolf					
chili hot dog sauce	about ⅙ c	?	2	?	44

□ **SEAFOOD & SEAFOOD PRODUCTS**
See also DINNERS, FROZEN; ENTREES &
MAIN COURSES, FROZEN

	Portion	Chol (mg)	Total Fat (g)	Satur'd Fat (g)	Total Calor

Finfish

ahi *See* tuna: yellowfin, *below*
aku *See* tuna: skipjack, *below*
anchovy, European
| raw | 3 oz | ? | 4 | 1 | 111 |
| canned in oil, drained solids | 5 | ? | 2 | tr | 42 |

bass, freshwater
mixed species, raw	3 oz	58	3	1	97
striped, raw	3 oz	68	2	tr	82
bluefish, raw	3 oz	50	4	1	105
burbot, raw	3 oz	51	1	tr	76
butterfish, raw	3 oz	55	7	?	124

carp
| raw | 3 oz | 56 | 5 | 1 | 108 |
| baked, broiled, micro-waved | 3 oz | 72 | 6 | 1 | 138 |

catfish
channel
| raw | 3 oz | 49 | 4 | 1 | 99 |
| breaded & fried | 3 oz | 69 | 11 | 3 | 194 |

ocean *See* wolffish, *below*
chub *See* cisco: smoked, *below*
cisco
raw	3 oz	?	2	tr	84
smoked	1 oz	9	3	tr	50
	3 oz	27	10	1	151

cod
Atlantic
raw	3 oz	37	1	tr	70
baked, broiled, micro-waved	3 oz	47	1	tr	89
canned, solids & liquids	3 oz	47	1	tr	89
dried & salted	1 oz	42	1	tr	81
	3 oz	129	2	tr	246
Pacific, raw	3 oz	31	1	tr	70

croaker, Atlantic
raw	3 oz	52	3	1	89
breaded & fried	3 oz	71	11	3	188
cusk, raw	3 oz	35	1	?	74

dogfish *See* shark, *below*
| dolphin fish, raw | 3 oz | 62 | 1 | tr | 73 |
| drum, freshwater, raw | 3 oz | 54 | 4 | 1 | 101 |
eel, mixed species
| raw | 3 oz | 107 | 10 | 2 | 156 |

	Portion	Chol (mg)	Total Fat (g)	Satur'd Fat (g)	Total Calor
eel, mixed species *(cont.)*					
baked, broiled, micro-waved	3 oz	137	13	3	200
flatfish					
raw	3 oz	41	1	tr	78
baked, broiled, micro-waved	3 oz	58	1	tr	99
flounder *See* flatfish, *above*					
grouper, mixed species					
raw	3 oz	31	1	tr	78
baked, broiled, micro-waved	3 oz	40	1	tr	100
haddock					
raw	3 oz	49	1	tr	74
baked, broiled, micro-waved	3 oz	63	1	tr	95
smoked	1 oz	21	tr	tr	33
	3 oz	65	1	tr	99
hake *See* whiting, *below*					
halibut					
Atlantic or Pacific					
raw	3 oz	27	2	tr	93
baked, broiled, micro-waved	3 oz	35	2	tr	119
Greenland, raw	3 oz	39	12	2	158
herring					
Atlantic					
raw	3 oz	51	8	2	134
baked, broiled, micro-waved	3 oz	65	10	2	172
canned *See* sardine: Atlantic, *below*					
kippered	1.4 oz	33	5	1	87
pickled	½ oz	2	3	tr	39
lake *See* cisco, *above*					
Pacific, raw	3 oz	65	12	3	166
ling, raw	3 oz	?	1	?	74
lingcod, raw	3 oz	44	1	tr	72
lox *See* salmon: chinook, smoked, *below*					
mackerel					
Atlantic					
raw	3 oz	60	12	3	174
baked, broiled, micro-waved	3 oz	64	15	4	223
jack, canned, drained solids	1 c	150	12	3	296
king, raw	3 oz	45	2	tr	89
Pacific & jack, mixed species, raw	3 oz	40	7	2	133
Spanish					
raw	3 oz	65	5	2	118

	Portion	Chol (mg)	Total Fat (g)	Satur'd Fat (g)	Total Calor
baked, broiled, micro-waved	3 oz	62	5	2	134
mahimahi *See* dolphin fish, *above*					
milkfish, raw	3 oz	44	6	?	126
monkfish, raw	3 oz	21	1	?	64
mullet, striped					
raw	3 oz	42	3	1	99
baked, broiled, micro-waved	3 oz	54	4	1	127
ocean perch, Atlantic					
raw	3 oz	36	1	tr	80
baked, broiled, micro-waved	3 oz	46	2	tr	103
perch, mixed species					
raw	3 oz	76	1	tr	77
baked, broiled, micro-waved	3 oz	98	1	tr	99
pike					
northern					
raw	3 oz	33	1	tr	75
baked, broiled, micro-waved	3 oz	43	1	tr	96
walleye, raw	3 oz	73	1	tr	79
pollock					
Atlantic, raw	3 oz	60	1	tr	78
walleye					
raw	3 oz	61	1	tr	68
baked, broiled, micro-waved	3 oz	82	1	tr	96
pompano, Florida					
raw	3 oz	43	8	3	140
baked, broiled, micro-waved	3 oz	54	10	4	179
porgy *See* scup, *below*					
pout, ocean, raw	3 oz	44	1	tr	67
redfish *See* ocean perch, *above*					
rockfish, Pacific, mixed species					
raw	3 oz	29	1	tr	80
baked, broiled, micro-waved	3 oz	38	2	tr	103
roughy, orange, raw	3 oz	17	6	tr	107
sablefish					
raw	3 oz	42	13	3	166
smoked	1 oz	18	6	1	72
salmon					
Atlantic, raw	3 oz	47	5	1	121
chinook					
raw	3 oz	56	9	2	153
smoked	1 oz	7	1	tr	33
	3 oz	20	4	1	99

	Portion	Chol (mg)	Total Fat (g)	Satur'd Fat (g)	Total Calor
salmon *(cont.)*					
chum					
raw	3 oz	63	3	1	102
canned, drained solids	3 oz	33	5	1	120
w/bone	13 oz	144	20	5	521
coho					
raw	3 oz	33	5	1	124
boiled, poached, steamed	3 oz	42	6	1	157
pink					
raw	3 oz	44	3	tr	99
canned, solids w/bone	3 oz	?	5	1	118
& liquid	16 oz	?	27	7	631
red *See* salmon: sockeye, *below*					
sockeye					
raw	3 oz	53	7	1	143
baked, broiled, microwaved	3 oz	74	9	2	183
canned, drained solids	3 oz	37	6	1	130
w/bone	13 oz	161	27	6	566
sardine					
Atlantic, canned in oil, drained solids w/bone	2 sardines = 0.8 oz	34	3	tr	50
	3.2 oz	131	11	1	192
Pacific, canned in tomato sauce, drained solids	1 sardine = 1.3 oz	23	5	1	68
w/bone	13 oz	225	44	11	658
scrod *See* cod: Atlantic, *above*					
scup, raw	3 oz	?	2	?	89
sea bass, mixed species					
raw	3 oz	35	2	tr	82
baked, broiled, microwaved	3 oz	45	2	1	105
sea trout, mixed species, raw	3 oz	71	3	1	88
shad, American, raw	3 oz	?	12	?	167
shark, mixed species					
raw	3 oz	43	4	1	111
batter-dipped & fried	3 oz	50	12	3	194
sheepshead					
raw	3 oz	?	2	1	92
baked, broiled, microwaved	3 oz	?	1	tr	107
smelt, rainbow					
raw	3 oz	60	2	tr	83
baked, broiled, microwaved	3 oz	76	3	tr	106
snapper, mixed species					
raw	3 oz	31	1	tr	85
baked, broiled, microwaved	3 oz	40	1	tr	109
sole *See* flatfish, *above*					

	Portion	Chol (mg)	Total Fat (g)	Satur'd Fat (g)	Total Calor
spot, raw	3 oz	?	4	1	105
sturgeon, mixed species					
raw	3 oz	?	3	1	90
baked, broiled, micro-waved	3 oz	?	4	1	115
smoked	1 oz	?	1	tr	48
	3 oz	?	4	1	147
sucker, white, raw	3 oz	35	2	tr	79
sunfish, pumpkinseed, raw	3 oz	57	1	tr	76
swordfish					
raw	3 oz	33	3	1	103
baked, broiled, micro-waved	3 oz	43	4	1	132
tilefish					
raw	3 oz	?	2	tr	81
baked, broiled, micro-waved	3 oz	?	4	1	125
trout					
mixed species, raw	3 oz	49	6	1	126
rainbow					
raw	3 oz	48	3	1	100
baked, broiled, micro-waved	3 oz	62	4	1	129
tuna					
bluefin					
raw	3 oz	32	4	1	122
baked, broiled, micro-waved	3 oz	42	5	1	157
light, canned					
in soybean oil, drained	3 oz	15	7	1	169
solids	6 oz	30	14	3	339
in water, drained solids	3 oz	?	tr	tr	111
	5.8 oz	?	1	tr	216
skipjack, raw	3 oz	40	1	tr	88
white, canned					
in soybean oil, drained	3 oz	26	7	?	158
solids	6.3 oz	55	14	?	331
in water, drained solids	3 oz	35	2	1	116
	6.1 oz	72	4	1	234
yellowfin, raw	3 oz	38	1	tr	92
turbot					
domestic See halibut: Greenland, above					
European, raw	3 oz	?	3	?	81
whitefish, mixed species					
raw	3 oz	51	5	1	114
smoked	1 oz	9	tr	tr	30
	3 oz	28	1	tr	92
whiting, mixed species					
raw	3 oz	57	1	tr	77
baked, broiled, micro-waved	3 oz	71	1	tr	98

	Portion	Chol (mg)	Total Fat (g)	Satur'd Fat (g)	Total Calor
wolffish, Atlantic, raw	3 oz	39	2	tr	82
yellowtail, mixed species, raw	3 oz	?	4	?	124

Shellfish

abalone, mixed species					
raw	3 oz	72	1	tr	89
fried	3 oz	80	6	1	161
clams, mixed species					
raw	3 oz	29	1	tr	63
	9 large (50/qt) or 20 small (110/qt)	60	2	tr	133
boiled, poached, steamed	3 oz	57	2	tr	126
	20 small (110/qt)	60	2	tr	133
breaded & fried	3 oz	52	9	2	171
	20 small (110/qt)	115	21	5	379
canned, drained solids	3 oz	57	2	tr	126
	1 c	107	3	tr	236
canned, liquid	3 oz	?	tr	?	2
	1 c	?	tr	?	6
crab					
Alaska king					
raw	3 oz	35	1	?	71
	1 leg = 1 lb	72	1	?	144
boiled, poached, steamed	3 oz	45	1	tr	82
	1 leg = 1 lb	72	2	tr	129
blue					
raw	1 crab = ⅓ lb	16	tr	tr	18
	3 oz	66	1	tr	74
boiled, poached, steamed	3 oz	85	2	tr	87
	1 c not packed	135	2	tr	138
canned, dry pack or drained solids of wet pack	3 oz	76	1	tr	84
	1 c not packed	120	2	tr	133
Dungeness, raw	3 oz	50	1	tr	73
	1 crab = 1½ lb	97	2	tr	140
queen, raw	3 oz	47	1	tr	76
crayfish, mixed species					
raw	3 oz	118	1	tr	76
boiled, poached, steamed	3 oz	151	1	tr	97

	Portion	Chol (mg)	Total Fat (g)	Satur'd Fat (g)	Total Calor
cuttlefish, mixed species, raw	3 oz	95	1	tr	67
lobster, northern					
raw	3 oz	81	1	?	77
	1 lobster = 1½ lb	143	1	?	136
boiled, poached, steamed	3 oz	61	1	tr	83
	1 c	104	1	tr	142
mussels, blue					
raw	3 oz	24	2	tr	73
	1 c	42	3	1	129
boiled, poached, steamed	3 oz	48	4	1	147
octopus, common, raw	3 oz	41	1	tr	70
oysters					
eastern					
raw	6 medium (70/qt)	46	2	1	58
	1 c	136	6	2	170
boiled, poached, steamed	6 medium (70/qt)	46	2	1	58
	3 oz	93	4	1	117
breaded & fried	3 oz	69	11	3	167
	6 medium (70/qt)	72	11	3	173
canned, solids & liquids	3 oz	46	2	1	58
	1 c	136	6	2	170
Pacific, raw	1 medium (20/qt)	?	1	tr	41
	3 oz	?	2	tr	69
scallops, mixed species					
raw	2 large (30/ lb) or 5 small (75/ lb)	10	tr	tr	26
	3 oz	28	1	tr	75
breaded & fried	2 large (30/ lb)	19	3	1	67
shrimp, mixed species					
raw	4 large (32/ lb)	43	tr	tr	30
	3 oz	130	1	tr	90
boiled, poached, steamed	4 large (32/ lb)	43	tr	tr	22
	3 oz	166	1	tr	84
breaded & fried	4 large (32/ lb)	53	4	1	73
	3 oz	150	10	2	206
canned, dry pack or	3 oz	147	2	tr	102
drained solids of wet pack	1 c	222	3	tr	154

snail, sea *See* whelk, *below*

	Portion	Chol (mg)	Total Fat (g)	Satur'd Fat (g)	Total Calor
spiny lobster, mixed species, raw	3 oz	60	1	tr	95
	1 lobster = 2 lb	146	3	tr	233
squid, mixed species					
raw	3 oz	198	1	tr	78
fried	3 oz	221	6	2	149
whelk					
raw	3 oz	55	tr	tr	117
boiled, poached, steamed	3 oz	110	1	tr	233

Seafood Products

	Portion	Chol (mg)	Total Fat (g)	Satur'd Fat (g)	Total Calor
caviar, black & red, granular	1 T	94	3	?	40
	1 oz	165	5	?	71
crab cakes (blue crab)	2.1 oz	90	6	1	93
fish sticks (walleye pollock), frozen, reheated	1 oz	31	3	1	76
gefilte fish, commercial, sweet recipe w/broth	1½ oz	12	1	tr	35
imitation seafood made from surimi					
crab, Alaska king	3 oz	17	1	?	87
scallops, mixed species	3 oz	18	tr	?	84
shrimp, mixed species	3 oz	31	1	?	86
roe, mixed species, raw	1 oz	105	2	tr	39
surimi (processed from walleye pollock)	1 oz	8	tr	?	28
	3 oz	25	1	?	84
tuna salad	3 oz	11	8	1	159
	1 c	27	19	3	383

▪ BRAND NAME

	Portion	Chol (mg)	Total Fat (g)	Satur'd Fat (g)	Total Calor
Featherweight					
salmon, pink	3⅞ oz	?	6	?	140
sardines					
canned in oil	1⅞ oz	?	6	?	109
canned in tomato	1⅞ oz	?	6	?	?
canned in water	1⅞ oz	?	6	?	109
tuna, light chunk	6½ oz	?	3	?	210
Fresh Chef					
seafood pasta salad	4¼ oz	?	17	?	240
Health Valley					
Best of Sea Food tuna	6½ oz	?	3	?	180
No Salt Diet tuna	6½ oz	?	3	?	200
Rokeach					
Natural Broth gefilte fish	1 ball = 2 oz	?	1	?	46
Old Vienna gefilte fish	1 ball = 2.6 oz	?	2	?	68

	Portion	Chol (mg)	Total Fat (g)	Satur'd Fat (g)	Total Calor
Old Vienna whitefish & pike gefilte fish	1 ball = 2.6 oz	?	1	?	70
whitefish & pike gefilte fish in jellied broth	1 ball = 2 oz	?	1	?	46

❑ SEASONINGS

See also BREADCRUMBS, CROUTONS, STUFFINGS, & SEASONED COATINGS; SAUCES, GRAVIES, & CONDIMENTS; VEGETABLES, PLAIN & PREPARED

NOTE: Most spices & herbs for which values are available contain less than ½ gram of fat, no cholesterol, and fewer than 10 calories per teaspoon. The following are exceptions.

	Portion	Chol (mg)	Total Fat (g)	Satur'd Fat (g)	Total Calor
mace, ground	1 t	0	1	tr	8
mustard powder	1 t	0	1	?	9
mustard seed, yellow	1 t	0	1	tr	15
nutmeg, ground	1 t	0	1	1	12
poppy seed	1 t	0	1	tr	15

▪ BRAND NAME

Featherweight

	Portion	Chol (mg)	Total Fat (g)	Satur'd Fat (g)	Total Calor
garlic salt substitute	¼ t	?	0	0	0
salt substitute	¼ t	?	0	?	0
seasoned salt substitute	¼ t	?	0	0	0
Health Valley					
all purpose	1 t	0	1	?	11
chicken	1 t	0	tr	?	8
fish	1 t	0	tr	?	11
steak/ham	1 t	0	tr	?	6
vegetable	1 t	0	tr	?	13
Kikkoman					
teriyaki baste & glaze	1 t	0	tr	?	9
Ortega					
mild taco meat seasoning	1 oz	0	1	0	90
Shake 'n Bake Seasoning Mixture					
Italian herb recipe	¼ pouch	0	1	?	80
Original Recipe					
for chicken	¼ pouch	0	2	?	80
for fish	¼ pouch	0	1	?	70
for pork	¼ pouch	0	1	?	80
for pork barbecue	¼ pouch	0	2	?	80

	Portion	Chol (mg)	Total Fat (g)	Satur'd Fat (g)	Total Calor

☐ SEEDS & SEED-BASED BUTTERS, FLOURS, & MEALS

See also NUTS & NUT-BASED BUTTERS, FLOURS, MEALS, MILKS, PASTES, & POWDERS

	Portion	Chol (mg)	Total Fat (g)	Satur'd Fat (g)	Total Calor
alfalfa seeds, sprouted, raw	1 c	0	tr	tr	10
breadfruit seeds					
raw	1 oz	0	2	tr	54
boiled	1 oz	0	1	tr	48
roasted	1 oz	0	1	tr	59
breadnuttree seeds					
raw	1 oz	0	tr	tr	62
dried	1 oz	0	tr	tr	104
chia seeds, dried	1 oz	0	7	3	134
cottonseed flour					
partially defatted	1 T	0	tr	tr	18
	1 c	0	6	1	337
low-fat	1 oz	0	tr	tr	94
cottonseed kernels, roasted	1 T	0	4	1	51
	1 c	0	54	14	754
cottonseed meal, partially defatted	1 oz	0	1	tr	104
lotus seeds					
raw	1 oz	0	tr	tr	25
dried	1 oz	0	1	tr	94
	1 c	0	1	tr	106
pumpkin & squash seeds					
whole, roasted	1 oz	0	6	1	127
	1 c	0	12	2	285
kernels					
dried	1 oz	0	13	2	154
	1 c	0	63	12	747
roasted	1 oz	0	12	2	148
	1 c	0	96	18	1,184
ramons *See* breadnuttree seeds, *above*					
safflower seed kernels, dried	1 oz	0	11	1	147
safflower seed meal, partially defatted	1 oz	0	1	tr	97
sesame butter					
paste	1 oz	0	14	2	169
	1 T	0	8	1	95
tahini					
from raw & stone-ground kernels	1 oz	0	14	2	162
	1 T	0	7	1	86
from roasted & toasted kernels	1 oz	0	15	2	169
	1 T	0	8	1	89

	Portion	Chol (mg)	Total Fat (g)	Satur'd Fat (g)	Total Calor
from unroasted kernels	1 oz	0	16	2	173
	1 T	0	8	1	85
sesame flour					
high-fat	1 oz	0	11	1	149
partially defatted	1 oz	0	3	tr	109
low-fat	1 oz	0	1	tr	95
sesame meal, partially defatted	1 oz	0	14	2	161
sesame seeds					
whole					
dried	1 T	0	4	1	52
	1 c	0	72	10	825
roasted & toasted kernels	1 oz	0	14	2	161
dried	1 T	0	4	1	47
	1 c	0	82	12	882
toasted	1 oz	0	14	2	161
sisymbrium sp. seeds,	1 oz	0	1	tr	90
whole, dried	1 c	0	3	1	235
squash seeds *See* pumpkin & squash seeds, *above*					
sunflower seed butter	1 T	0	8	1	93
sunflower seed flour, partially defatted	1 T	0	tr	tr	16
	1 c	0	1	tr	261
sunflower seed kernels					
dried	1 oz	0	14	1	162
	1 c	0	71	7	821
dry roasted	1 oz	0	14	1	165
	1 c	0	64	7	745
oil roasted	1 oz	0	16	2	175
	1 c	0	78	8	830
toasted	1 oz	0	16	2	176
	1 c	0	76	8	829
tahini *See* sesame butter: tahini, *above*					
watermelon seed kernels,	1 oz	0	13	3	158
dried	1 c	0	51	11	602

▪ BRAND NAME

Arrowhead Mills

alfalfa seeds, sprouted	1 c	0	1	?	40
amaranth seeds	2 oz	0	3	?	200
flax seeds	1 oz	0	10	?	140
sesame seeds, hulled or whole	1 oz	0	14	?	160
sesame tahini, chemical-free	1 oz	0	17	?	170
sunflower seeds, hulled	1 oz	0	13	?	160

	Portion	Chol (mg)	Total Fat (g)	Satur'd Fat (g)	Total Calor
Planters					
sunflower seeds	1 oz	0	14	2	160

☐ SHERBETS *See* DESSERTS, FROZEN

☐ SHORTENINGS *See* FATS, OILS, & SHORTENINGS

☐ SNACKS
See also CRACKERS

	Portion	Chol (mg)	Total Fat (g)	Satur'd Fat (g)	Total Calor
cheese puffs	1 oz	1	10	?	159
cheese straws	4	?	7	?	109
corn chips	1 oz	0	9	1	155
popcorn					
air-popped	1 c	0	tr	tr	30
popped in vegetable oil	1 c	0	3	1	55
sugar-syrup-coated	1 c	0	1	tr	135
potato chips	10	0	7	2	105
made from dried potatoes	1 oz	0	13	4	164
potato sticks	1 oz	0	10	3	148
	½ c	0	6	2	94
pretzels					
stick	10	0	tr	tr	10
twisted, Dutch	1	0	1	tr	65
twisted, thin	10	0	2	tr	240
tortilla chips	1 oz	0	7	?	139

■ BRAND NAME

	Portion	Chol (mg)	Total Fat (g)	Satur'd Fat (g)	Total Calor
Arrowhead Mills					
popcorn, unpopped	2 oz	0	3	?	210
Cornnuts					
Original or unsalted	1 oz	0	4	?	120
barbecue or nacho cheese	1 oz	0	4	?	110
Del Monte					
pineapple nuggets	0.9 oz	?	0	?	90
Sierra trail mix	0.9 oz	?	7	?	130
tropical fruit mix	0.9 oz	?	1	?	90
yogurt raisins, plain or strawberry	0.9 oz	?	5	?	120

	Portion	Chol (mg)	Total Fat (g)	Satur'd Fat (g)	Total Calor
Featherweight					
cheese curls	1 oz	?	9	?	150
corn chips	1 oz	?	11	?	170
nacho cheese chips	1 oz	?	8	?	150
potato chips	1 oz	?	11	?	160
pretzels	3	?	0	?	20
round tortilla chips	1 oz	?	8	?	150
Health Valley					
CORN CHIPS					
corn chips, regular or no salt	1 oz	0	11	?	160
cheese corn chips					
regular	1 oz	2	11	?	160
no salt	1 oz	2	10	?	160
POTATO CHIPS					
Country Chips, regular or no salt	1 oz	0	11	?	160
Country Ripples, regular or no salt	1 oz	0	11	?	160
potato chips, regular or no salt	1 oz	0	11	?	160
potato chips, dip, regular or no salt	1 oz	0	11	?	160
SNACK PUFFS					
Carrot Lites	17	0	1	?	70
Cheddar Lites					
regular or no salt	17	tr	2	?	40
w/green onion	17	0	1	?	40
TORTILLA CHIPS					
Buenitos: regular, no salt, or nacho cheese & chili	1 oz	1	8	?	150
Mister Salty Pretzels					
butter-flavored sticks	90	?	1	?	110
Dutch	2	?	1	?	110
Junior	29	?	2	?	110
Mini Mix	23	?	1	?	110
sticks	90	?	1	?	110
Veri-Thin sticks	45	?	1	?	110
Nabisco					
DOO DADS					
Original	1 oz or ½ c	?	6	?	140
cheddar & herb	1 oz or ½ c	?	6	?	140
Zesty cheese	1 oz or ½ c	?	6	?	140

	Portion	Chol (mg)	Total Fat (g)	Satur'd Fat (g)	Total Calor
GREAT CRISPS!					
cheese & chive	9	?	4	?	70
French onion	7	?	4	?	70
Italian	9	?	4	?	70
nacho	8	?	4	?	70
Real bacon	9	?	4	?	70
savory garlic	8	?	3	?	70
sesame	9	?	4	?	70
sour cream & onion	8	?	4	?	70
tomato & celery	9	?	4	?	70
NIPS					
Real cheddar cheese	13	?	3	?	70
pizza	20	?	3	?	70
taco	14	?	4	?	70
Pepperidge Farm *SNACK STICKS*					
Original	8	?	5	?	130
cheese	8	?	6	?	130
sesame	8	?	5	?	130
TINY GOLDFISH					
Original	45	?	7	?	140
cheddar cheese	45	?	6	?	140
Planters					
Cheez Balls	1 oz	5	11	2	160
Cheez Curls	1 oz	5	11	2	160
corn chips	1 oz	0	10	2	160
Fruit 'n Nut Mix	1 oz	0	9	2	150
popcorn	3 c popped	0	0	0	20
microwave, butter	3 c popped	0	10	1	140
microwave, natural	3 c popped	0	9	1	140
Potato Crunchies	1¼ oz	0	11	2	190
pretzels	1 oz	0	1	?	110
round toast crackers	4	0	7	2	140
sour cream & onion puffs	1 oz	0	10	2	160
square cheese crackers	4	0	7	1	140
Rokeach					
Dutch pretzels	1 oz	?	0	0	110

❏ SOUPS, PREPARED

Canned

	Portion	Chol (mg)	Total Fat (g)	Satur'd Fat (g)	Total Calor
asparagus, cream of, condensed	1 can = 10¾ oz	12	10	3	210

	Portion	Chol (mg)	Total Fat (g)	Satur'd Fat (g)	Total Calor
prepared w/water	1 c	5	4	1	87
prepared w/whole milk	1 c	22	8	3	161
	1 can	54	20	8	392
bean, black, condensed	1 can = 11 oz	0	4	1	285
prepared w/water	1 c	0	2	tr	116
bean w/bacon, condensed	1 can = 11½ oz	6	14	4	420
prepared w/water	1 c	3	6	2	173
bean w/frankfurter, condensed	1 can = 11¼ oz	29	17	5	454
prepared w/water	1 c	12	7	2	187
bean w/ham, chunky, ready-to-serve	1 c	22	9	3	231
	1 can = 19¼ oz	49	19	7	519
beef, chunky, ready-to-serve	1 c	14	5	3	171
	1 can = 19 oz	32	12	6	383
beef broth or bouillon, ready-to-serve	1 c	tr	1	tr	16
	1 can = 14 oz	1	1	tr	27
beef mushroom, condensed	1 can = 10¾ oz	15	7	4	?
prepared w/water	1 c	7	3	1	?
beef noodle, condensed	1 can = 10¾ oz	12	7	3	204
prepared w/water	1 c	5	3	1	84
celery, cream of, condensed	1 can = 10¾ oz	34	14	3	219
prepared w/water	1 c	15	6	1	90
prepared w/whole milk	1 c	32	10	4	165
	1 can	78	24	10	400
cheese, condensed	1 can = 11 oz	72	25	16	377
prepared w/water	1 c	30	10	7	155
prepared w/whole milk	1 c	48	15	9	230
	1 can	116	35	22	558
chicken, chunky, ready-to-serve	1 c	30	7	2	178
	1 can = 10¾ oz	37	8	2	216
chicken, cream of, condensed	1 can = 10¾ oz	24	18	5	283
prepared w/water	1 c	10	7	2	116
prepared w/whole milk	1 c	27	11	5	191
	1 can	66	28	11	464
chicken & dumplings, condensed	1 can = 10½ oz	80	13	3	236
prepared w/water	1 c	34	6	1	97

	Portion	Chol (mg)	Total Fat (g)	Satur'd Fat (g)	Total Calor
chicken broth, condensed	1 can = 10¾ oz	3	3	1	94
prepared w/water	1 c	1	1	tr	39
chicken gumbo, condensed	1 can = 10¾ oz	9	3	1	137
prepared w/water	1 c	5	1	tr	56
chicken mushroom, condensed	1 can = 10¾ oz	24	22	6	?
prepared w/water	1 c	10	9	2	?
chicken noodle					
chunky, ready-to-serve	1 c	18	6	1	?
	1 can = 19 oz	40	13	3	?
condensed	1 can = 10½ oz	15	6	1	182
prepared w/water	1 c	7	2	1	75
chicken noodle w/meatballs, ready-to-serve	1 c	10	4	1	99
	1 can = 20 oz	23	8	2	227
chicken rice					
chunky, ready-to-serve	1 c	12	3	1	127
	1 can = 19 oz	27	7	2	286
condensed	1 can = 10½ oz	15	5	1	146
prepared w/water	1 c	7	2	tr	60
chicken vegetable					
chunky, ready-to-serve	1 c	17	5	1	167
	1 can = 19 oz	38	11	3	374
condensed	1 can = 10½ oz	21	7	2	181
prepared w/water	1 c	10	3	1	74
chili beef, condensed	1 can = 11¼ oz	32	16	8	411
prepared w/water	1 c	12	7	3	169
clam chowder (Manhattan)					
chunky, ready-to-serve	1 c	14	3	2	133
	1 can = 19 oz	32	8	5	299
condensed	1 can = 10¾ oz	6	5	1	187
prepared w/water	1 c	2	2	tr	78
clam chowder (New England), condensed	1 can = 10¾ oz	12	6	1	214
prepared w/water	1 c	5	3	tr	95
prepared w/whole milk	1 c	22	7	3	163
	1 can	54	16	7	396
consommé w/gelatin, condensed	1 can = 10½ oz	0	0	0	71
prepared w/water	1 c	0	0	0	29

	Portion	Chol (mg)	Total Fat (g)	Satur'd Fat (g)	Total Calor
crab, ready-to-serve	1 c	10	2	tr	76
	1 can = 13 oz	10	2	1	114
escarole, ready-to-serve	1 c	2	2	1	27
	1 can = 19½ oz	6	4	1	61
gazpacho, ready-to-serve	1 c	0	2	tr	57
	1 can = 13 oz	0	3	tr	87
lentil w/ham, ready-to-serve	1 c	7	3	1	140
	1 can = 20 oz	17	6	3	320
minestrone					
chunky, ready-to-serve	1 c	5	3	1	127
	1 can = 19 oz	11	6	3	285
condensed	1 can = 10½ oz	3	6	1	202
prepared w/water	1 c	2	3	1	83
mushroom, cream of, condensed	1 can = 10¾ oz	3	23	6	313
prepared w/water	1 c	2	9	2	129
prepared w/whole milk	1 c	20	14	5	203
	1 can	48	33	12	494
mushroom barley, condensed	1 can = 10¾ oz	0	5	1	?
prepared w/water	1 c	0	2	tr	?
mushroom w/beef stock, condensed	1 can = 10¾ oz	18	10	4	208
prepared w/water	1 c	7	4	2	85
onion, condensed	1 can = 10½ oz	0	4	1	138
prepared w/water	1 c	0	2	tr	57
onion, cream of, condensed	1 can = 10¾ oz	37	13	4	?
prepared w/water	1 c	15	5	1	?
prepared w/whole milk	1 c	32	9	4	?
	1 can	78	23	10	?
oyster stew, condensed	1 can = 10½ oz	33	9	6	144
prepared w/water	1 c	14	4	3	59
prepared w/whole milk	1 c	32	8	5	134
	1 can	77	19	12	325
pea, green, condensed	1 can = 11¼ oz	0	7	3	398
prepared w/water	1 c	0	3	1	164
prepared w/whole milk	1 c	18	7	4	239
	1 can	43	17	10	579
pea, split, w/ham					
chunky, ready-to-serve	1 c	7	4	2	184
	1 can = 19 oz	16	9	4	413

	Portion	Chol (mg)	Total Fat (g)	Satur'd Fat (g)	Total Calor
condensed	1 can = 11½ oz	20	11	4	459
prepared w/water	1 c	8	4	2	189
pepperpot, condensed	1 can = 10½ oz	24	11	5	251
prepared w/water	1 c	10	5	2	103
potato, cream of, condensed	1 can = 10¾ oz	15	6	3	178
prepared w/water	1 c	5	2	1	73
prepared w/whole milk	1 c	22	6	4	148
	1 can	54	16	9	360
Scotch broth, condensed	1 can = 10½ oz	12	6	3	195
prepared w/water	1 c	5	3	1	80
shrimp, cream of, condensed	1 can = 10¾ oz	40	13	8	219
prepared w/water	1 c	17	5	3	90
prepared w/whole milk	1 c	35	9	6	165
	1 can	84	23	14	400
stockpot, condensed	1 can = 11 oz	9	9	2	242
prepared w/water	1 c	5	4	1	100
tomato, condensed	1 can = 10¾ oz	0	5	1	208
prepared w/water	1 c	0	2	tr	86
prepared w/whole milk	1 c	17	6	3	160
	1 can	42	15	7	389
tomato beef w/noodle, condensed	1 can = 10¾ oz	9	10	4	341
prepared w/water	1 c	5	4	2	140
tomato bisque, condensed	1 can = 11 oz	11	6	1	300
prepared w/water	1 c	4	3	1	123
prepared w/whole milk	1 c	22	7	3	198
	1 can	53	16	8	481
tomato rice, condensed	1 can = 11 oz	3	7	1	291
prepared w/water	1 c	2	3	1	120
turkey, chunky, ready-to-serve	1 c	9	4	1	136
	1 can = 18¾ oz	21	10	3	306
turkey noodle, condensed	1 can = 10¾ oz	12	5	1	168
prepared w/water	1 c	5	2	1	69
turkey vegetable, condensed	1 can = 10½ oz	3	7	2	179
prepared w/water	1 c	2	3	1	74

	Portion	Chol (mg)	Total Fat (g)	Satur'd Fat (g)	Total Calor
vegetable, chunky, ready-to-serve	1 c	0	4	1	122
	1 can = 19 oz	0	8	1	274
vegetable, vegetarian, condensed	1 can = 10½ oz	0	5	1	176
prepared w/water	1 c	0	2	tr	72
vegetable w/beef, condensed	1 can = 10¾ oz	12	5	2	192
prepared w/water	1 c	5	2	1	79
vegetable w/beef broth, condensed	1 can = 10½ oz	6	5	1	197
prepared w/water	1 c	2	2	tr	81

Dehydrated

	Portion	Chol (mg)	Total Fat (g)	Satur'd Fat (g)	Total Calor
asparagus, cream of, prepared w/water	1 c	tr	2	tr	59
	39.7 oz	1	8	1	265
bean w/bacon, prepared w/water	1 c	3	2	1	105
beef broth or bouillon					
cubed	1 cube = 0.1 oz	tr	tr	tr	6
prepared w/water	1 c	1	1	tr	19
	6 fl oz	tr	1	tr	14
beef noodle, prepared w/water	1 c	2	1	tr	41
	6 fl oz	1	1	tr	30
cauliflower, prepared w/water	1 c	tr	2	tr	68
celery, cream of, prepared w/water	1 c	1	2	tr	63
chicken, cream of, prepared w/water	1 c	3	5	3	107
	6 fl oz	2	4	3	80
chicken broth or bouillon					
cubed	1 cube = 0.2 oz	1	tr	tr	9
prepared w/water	1 c	1	1	tr	21
	6 fl oz	1	1	tr	16
chicken noodle	1 pkt = 2.6 oz	10	6	1	257
	1 pkt = 0.4 oz	2	1	tr	38
prepared w/water	1 c	3	1	tr	53
chicken rice, prepared w/water	1 c	3	1	tr	60
chicken vegetable, prepared w/water	1 c	3	1	tr	49
	6 fl oz	2	1	tr	37
clam chowder (Manhattan)	1 c	0	2	tr	65
clam chowder (New England)	1 c	1	4	1	95

	Portion	Chol (mg)	Total Fat (g)	Satur'd Fat (g)	Total Calor
consommé, w/gelatin	1 c	0	tr	tr	17
added, prepared w/ water	39½ oz	0	tr	tr	77
leek, prepared w/water	1 c	3	2	1	71
	36 fl oz	11	9	5	319
minestrone, prepared w/	1 c	3	2	1	79
water	40.2 oz	11	8	4	358
mushroom	1 pkt regular = 2.6 oz	2	17	3	328
	1 pkt instant = 0.6 oz	0	4	1	74
prepared w/water	1 c	1	5	1	96
onion	1 pkt = 1.4 oz	2	2	1	115
	1 pkt = ¼ oz	0	tr	tr	21
prepared w/water	1 c	0	1	tr	28
oxtail, prepared w/water	1 c	3	3	1	71
	36 fl oz	11	11	6	318
pea, green or split	1 pkt = 4 oz	1	5	2	402
	1 pkt = 1 oz	0	1	tr	100
prepared w/water	1 c	3	2	tr	133
tomato (includes cream of tomato)	1 pkt = ¾ oz	1	2	1	77
prepared w/water	1 c	1	2	1	102
	6 fl oz	1	2	1	77
tomato vegetable (includes Italian vegetable & spring vegetable)	1 pkt = 1.4 oz	1	2	1	125
prepared w/water	1 c	tr	1	tr	55
	6 fl oz	tr	1	tr	41
vegetable, cream of, prepared w/water	1 c	0	6	1	105
	6 fl oz	0	4	1	79
vegetable beef, prepared w/water	1 c	1	1	1	53
	1 pkt = 40 oz	5	5	2	240

- **BRAND NAME**

Campbell
CHUNKY SOUPS, READY-TO-SERVE

bean w/ham, Old Fashioned	11 oz	?	9	?	290
	9⅝ oz	?	8	?	260
beef	10¾ oz	?	5	?	190
	9½ oz	?	4	?	170

	Portion	Chol (mg)	Total Fat (g)	Satur'd Fat (g)	Total Calor
chicken, Old Fashioned	9½ oz	?	4	?	150
chicken mushroom, creamy	10½ oz	?	26	?	320
	9⅜ oz	?	24	?	280
chicken noodle	9½ oz	?	6	?	180
chicken noodle w/mushroom	10¾ oz	?	7	?	200
chicken rice	9½ oz	?	4	?	140
chicken vegetable	9½ oz	?	6	?	170
chili beef	11 oz	?	7	?	290
	9¾ oz	?	6	?	260
clam chowder (Manhattan style)	10¾ oz	?	5	?	160
	9½ oz	?	4	?	150
clam chowder (New England style)	10¾ oz	?	17	?	290
	9½ oz	?	15	?	250
Fisherman chowder	10¾ oz	?	14	?	260
	9½ oz	?	13	?	230
minestrone	9½ oz	?	4	?	160
mushroom, creamy	10½ oz	?	22	?	260
	9⅜ oz	?	20	?	240
sirloin burger	10¾ oz	?	9	?	220
	9½ oz	?	8	?	200
split pea & ham	10¾ oz	?	6	?	230
	9½ oz	?	5	?	210
steak & potato	10¾ oz	?	5	?	200
	9½ oz	?	4	?	170
Stroganoff-style beef	10¾ oz	?	15	?	300
turkey vegetable	9⅜ oz	?	6	?	150
vegetable	10¾ oz	?	4	?	140
	9½ oz	?	4	?	130
vegetable, Mediterranean	9½ oz	?	5	?	160

CONDENSED SOUPS, AS PACKAGED

	Portion	Chol (mg)	Total Fat (g)	Satur'd Fat (g)	Total Calor
asparagus, cream of	4 oz	?	4	?	90
bean w/bacon	4 oz	?	5	?	150
beef broth (bouillon)	4 oz	?	0	?	16
beef noodle	4 oz	?	3	?	70
black bean	4 oz	?	2	?	110
celery, cream of	4 oz	?	7	?	100
cheddar cheese	4 oz	?	8	?	130
chicken, cream of	4 oz	?	7	?	110
chicken & dumplings	4 oz	?	3	?	80
chicken broth	4 oz	?	2	?	35
chicken gumbo	4 oz	?	2	?	60
chicken noodle	4 oz	?	2	?	70
chicken vegetable	4 oz	?	3	?	70
chicken w/rice	4 oz	?	2	?	60
chili beef	4 oz	?	5	?	130
clam chowder (Manhattan style)	4 oz	?	2	?	70
clam chowder (New England style)	4 oz	?	3	?	80

	Portion	Chol (mg)	Total Fat (g)	Satur'd Fat (g)	Total Calor
clam chowder *(cont.)*					
prepared w/whole milk	4 oz	?	7	?	150
French onion	4 oz	?	2	?	60
green pea	4 oz	?	3	?	160
minestrone	4 oz	?	2	?	80
mushroom, cream of	4 oz	?	7	?	100
mushroom, Golden	4 oz	?	3	?	80
nacho cheese	4 oz	?	8	?	100
noodles & ground beef	4 oz	?	4	?	90
onion, cream of	4 oz	?	5	?	100
prepared w/whole milk	4 oz	?	7	?	140
oyster stew	4 oz	?	5	?	80
prepared w/whole milk	4 oz	?	9	?	150
pepper pot	4 oz	?	4	?	90
potato, cream of	4 oz	?	3	?	70
prepared w/whole milk	4 oz	?	4	?	110
Scotch broth	4 oz	?	3	?	80
shrimp, cream of	4 oz	?	6	?	90
prepared w/whole milk	4 oz	?	10	?	160
Spanish-style vegetable (gazpacho)	4 oz	?	0	?	45
split pea w/ham & bacon	4 oz	?	4	?	160
tomato	4 oz	?	2	?	90
prepared w/whole milk	4 oz	?	6	?	160
tomato bisque	4 oz	?	3	?	120
tomato rice, Old Fashioned	4 oz	?	2	?	110
turkey noodle	4 oz	?	3	?	70
turkey vegetable	4 oz	?	3	?	70
vegetable	4 oz	?	2	?	90
vegetable, Old Fashioned	4 oz	?	2	?	60
vegetable, vegetarian	4 oz	?	2	?	90
vegetable beef	4 oz	?	2	?	70
won ton	4 oz	?	1	?	40
CREAMY NATURAL SOUPS, CONDENSED					
asparagus, prepared w/ whole milk	4 oz	?	9	?	170
potato, prepared w/whole milk	4 oz	?	11	?	190
DRY SOUP MIXES, AS PACKAGED					
cheddar cheese	1 oz	?	10	?	160
chicken noodle	1 oz	?	2	?	100
chicken rice	1 oz	?	2	?	90
noodle	1 oz	?	2	?	110
onion	½ oz	?	0	?	50
onion mushroom	½ oz	?	0	?	50
HOME COOKIN' SOUPS, READY-TO-SERVE					
chicken w/noodles	10¾ oz	?	4	?	140
country vegetable	10¾ oz	?	2	?	120
lentil	10¾ oz	?	1	?	170

	Portion	Chol (mg)	Total Fat (g)	Satur'd Fat (g)	Total Calor
minestrone	10¾ oz	?	3	?	140
split pea w/ham	10¾ oz	?	4	?	210
vegetable beef	10¾ oz	?	3	?	150

LOW-SODIUM SOUPS, READY-TO-SERVE

	Portion	Chol (mg)	Total Fat (g)	Satur'd Fat (g)	Total Calor
beef & mushroom, chunky	10¾ oz	?	7	?	210
chicken broth	10½ oz	?	2	?	40
chicken vegetable, chunky	10¾ oz	?	11	?	240
chicken w/noodles	10¾ oz	?	5	?	160
French onion	10½ oz	?	4	?	80
mushroom, cream of	10½ oz	?	14	?	200
split pea	10¾ oz	?	5	?	240
tomato w/tomato pieces	10½ oz	?	5	?	180
vegetable beef, chunky	10¾ oz	?	5	?	170

SEMICONDENSED SOUPS, AS PREPARED

	Portion	Chol (mg)	Total Fat (g)	Satur'd Fat (g)	Total Calor
bean w/ham, Old Fashioned	11 oz	?	7	?	220
chicken & noodles, Golden	11 oz	?	4	?	120
clam chowder (New England)	11 oz	?	4	?	130
prepared w/whole milk	11 oz	?	7	?	190
mushroom, savory cream of	11 oz	?	13	?	180
Tomato Royale	11 oz	?	3	?	180
vegetable, Old World	11 oz	?	4	?	130
vegetable beef & bacon, Burly	11 oz	?	5	?	160

College Inn

	Portion	Chol (mg)	Total Fat (g)	Satur'd Fat (g)	Total Calor
beef broth	1 c	?	0	?	18
chicken broth	1 c	?	3	?	35

Featherweight

	Portion	Chol (mg)	Total Fat (g)	Satur'd Fat (g)	Total Calor
bouillon, instant beef or chicken	1 t	?	1	0	18
chicken noodle	3¾ oz	?	2	?	60
mushroom	3¾ oz	?	2	0	50
tomato	3¾ oz	?	0	0	60
vegetable beef	3¾ oz	?	3	0	80

Health Valley

	Portion	Chol (mg)	Total Fat (g)	Satur'd Fat (g)	Total Calor
bean, regular or no salt	4 oz	0	3	?	115
beef broth, regular or no salt	4 oz	?	0	?	10
chicken broth, regular or no salt	4 oz	2	2	?	30
clam chowder, regular or no salt	4 oz	7	3	?	80
green split pea					
regular	4 oz	0	0	?	70
no salt	4 oz	0	1	?	80

	Portion	Chol (mg)	Total Fat (g)	Satur'd Fat (g)	Total Calor
lentil, regular or no salt	4 oz	0	4	?	80
minestrone, regular or no salt	4 oz	0	4	?	90
minestrone, chunky, regular or no salt	4 oz	0	1	?	70
mushroom, regular or no salt	4 oz	0	3	?	70
potato, regular or no salt	4 oz	0	2	?	70
tomato, regular or no salt	4 oz	0	2	?	60
vegetable, regular or no salt	4 oz	0	4	?	80
vegetable, chunky, regular or no salt	4 oz	0	2	?	70
vegetable chicken, chunky, regular or no salt	4 oz	12	7	?	120
Nissin					
CUP O'NOODLES					
beef	1 pkg = 1 c	?	14	?	290
chicken	1 pkg = 1 c	?	16	?	300
shrimp	1 pkg = 1 c	?	14	?	300
HEARTY CUP O'NOODLES					
cream of chicken	1 pkg = 1 c	?	17	?	330
OODLES OF NOODLES					
beef	1 pkg = 1 c	?	18	?	390
chicken	1 pkg = 1 c	?	18	?	400
QUICK 'N TENDER					
chicken	1 pkg = 1 c	?	28	?	600
STIR 'N READY					
chicken	1 pkg = 1 c	?	10	?	190
TWIN CUP O'NOODLES					
chicken	1 pkg = 1 c	?	7	?	150
Rokeach					
CONDENSED SOUPS					
celery, cream of	5 oz	0	4	?	90
mushroom, cream of	5 oz	?	10	?	150

	Portion	Chol (mg)	Total Fat (g)	Satur'd Fat (g)	Total Calor
tomato	5 oz	?	1	?	90
tomato w/rice	5 oz	0	5	?	160
vegetarian vegetable	5 oz	0	3	?	90
READY-TO-SERVE SOUPS					
borscht	8 fl oz	?	tr	?	96
creamed-style schav	1 c	?	?	?	12
Stouffer's Frozen Soups					
clam chowder (New England)	8 oz	?	11	?	200
spinach, cream of	8 oz	?	14	?	220
split pea w/ham	8¼ oz	?	3	?	200
Swanson					
beef broth	7¼ oz	?	1	?	20
chicken broth	7¼ oz	?	2	?	30

❑ SOUR CREAM *See* MILK, MILK SUBSTITUTES, & MILK PRODUCTS

❑ SOYBEANS & SOYBEAN PRODUCTS

Soybeans

boiled	½ c	0	8	1	149
dry roasted	½ c	0	19	3	387
mature seeds, sprouted					
raw	½ c	0	2	tr	45
steamed	½ c	0	2	tr	38
stir-fried	3½ oz	0	7	?	125
roasted	½ c	0	22	3	405

Soybean Products

fermented products					
miso	½ c	0	8	1	284
natto	½ c	0	10	1	187
tempeh	½ c	0	6	1	165
soy flour					
full-fat					
raw	½ c stirred	0	9	1	182
roasted	½ c stirred	0	9	1	184
low-fat	½ c stirred	0	3	tr	163
defatted	½ c stirred	0	1	tr	164
soy meal, defatted, raw	½ c	0	1	tr	206
soy milk, fluid	1 c	0	5	1	79

	Portion	Chol (mg)	Total Fat (g)	Satur'd Fat (g)	Total Calor
soy protein					
concentrate	1 oz	0	tr	tr	92
isolate	1 oz	0	1	tr	94
soy sauce					
made from hydrolyzed	1 T	0	tr	tr	7
vegetable protein	¼ c	0	tr	tr	24
made from soy (tamari)	1 T	0	tr	tr	11
	¼ c	0	tr	tr	35
made from soy & wheat	1 T	0	tr	tr	9
(shoyu)	¼ c	0	tr	tr	30
teriyaki sauce					
dehydrated	1 pkt = 1.6 oz	0	1	tr	130
prepared w/water	1 c	0	1	tr	131
ready-to-serve	1 T	0	0	0	15
	1 fl oz	0	0	0	30
tofu					
raw					
regular	4.1 oz	0	6	1	88
	½ c	0	6	1	94
firm	2.9 oz	0	7	1	118
	½ c	0	11	2	183
dried-frozen (koyadofu)	0.6 oz	0	5	1	82
fried	½ oz	0	3	tr	35
okara	½ c	0	1	tr	47
salted & fermented (fuyu)	0.4 oz	0	1	tr	13

• BRAND NAME

	Portion	Chol (mg)	Total Fat (g)	Satur'd Fat (g)	Total Calor
Arrowhead Mills					
soybean flakes	2 oz	0	11	?	250
soybeans	2 oz	0	10	?	230
soy flour	2 oz	0	11	?	250
tamari soy sauce	1 T	0	0	?	15
Chun King					
soy sauce	1 t	?	0	?	6
Fearn					
lecithin granules	2 level T	0	12	2	100
liquid lecithin					
regular	1 T	0	16	2	130
mint-flavored	1 T	0	16	2	113
natural soya powder	¼ c	0	5	1	100
soya granules	¼ c	0	tr	tr	140
soya protein isolate	¼ c	0	tr	tr	60
Health Valley					
Soy Moo soybean milk	8 fl oz	0	6	?	140
Tofu-Ya					
hard	4 oz	?	5	?	110
soft	4 oz	?	5	?	60

	Portion	Chol (mg)	Total Fat (g)	Satur'd Fat (g)	Total Calor
Kikkoman					
soy sauce, regular or lite	1 T	tr	tr	?	10
stir-fry sauce	1 t	0	tr	?	6
sweet & sour sauce	1 T	0	tr	?	18
teriyaki sauce	1 T	tr	tr	?	15

❑ SPICES *See* SEASONINGS

❑ STUFFINGS *See* BREADCRUMBS, CROUTONS, STUFFINGS, & SEASONED COATINGS

❑ SUGARS & SWEETENERS: HONEY, MOLASSES, SUGAR, SUGAR SUBSTITUTES, SYRUP, & TREACLE

	Portion	Chol (mg)	Total Fat (g)	Satur'd Fat (g)	Total Calor
HONEY					
honey	1 T	0	0	0	61
	5 T	0	0	0	306
MOLASSES					
first extraction, light	1 T	0	0	0	50
	5 T	0	0	0	252
second extraction, medium	1 T	0	0	0	46
	5 T	0	0	0	232
third extraction, blackstrap	1 T	0	0	0	43
	5 T	0	0	0	213
SUGAR					
brown	1 T	0	0	0	52
	5 T	0	0	0	364
maple	1 T	0	0	0	52
sugarcane juice	1 T	0	tr	?	16
white					
granulated	1 cube	0	0	0	24
	1 t	0	0	0	16
	1 T	0	0	0	46
	½ c	0	0	0	385
powdered	1 T	0	0	0	42
	9 T	0	0	0	385
SYRUP					
cane	1 T	0	0	0	53
	5 T	0	0	0	263

	Portion	Chol (mg)	Total Fat (g)	Satur'd Fat (g)	Total Calor
corn	1 T	0	0	0	57
	5 T	0	0	0	287
dark corn	1 T	0	0	0	60
maple	1 T	0	0	0	50
	5 T	0	0	0	252
maple, imitation	1 T	0	0	0	55
	5 T	0	0	0	275
sorghum, pancake	1 T	0	0	0	52
table blend, pancake					
cane & maple	1 T	0	0	0	50
mainly corn	1 T	0	0	0	57
	5 T	0	0	0	286
TREACLE					
black	1 T	0	0	0	53
	5 T	0	0	0	265

▪ BRAND NAME

Aunt Jemima
syrup	1 fl oz	?	0	0	103
Butter Lite syrup	1 fl oz	?	0	0	52
Lite syrup	1 fl oz	?	0	0	60

Brer Rabbit
molasses, light or dark	1 T	?	0	?	60

Diamond Crystal
sugar substitute	1 pkg	0	0	0	1

Equal
sugar substitute	1 pkg	0	0	0	4

Golden Griddle
syrup	1 T	0	0	0	50

Grandma's
molasses, gold or green label	1 T	0	0	0	70

Karo
corn syrup, dark or light	1 T	0	0	0	60
pancake syrup	1 T	0	0	0	60

Log Cabin
syrup	1 fl oz	0	0	0	104
buttered syrup	1 fl oz	2	1	tr	105
Country Kitchen syrup	1 fl oz	0	0	0	101
maple honey syrup	1 fl oz	0	0	0	106

NutraSweet
sugar substitute	1 pkg	0	0	0	4

Sprinkle Sweet
sugar substitute	⅛ t	0	0	0	2

	Portion	Chol (mg)	Total Fat (g)	Satur'd Fat (g)	Total Calor
Sugartwin					
sugar substitute					
white	1 pkg	0	0	0	3
white/brown	1 t	0	0	0	1
Sweet & Low					
sugar substitute	1 pkg	0	0	0	4
Sweet 10					
sugar substitute	⅛ t	0	0	0	0
Vermont Maid					
syrup	1 T	?	0	?	50

❑ **SYRUP** *See* SUGARS & SWEETENERS

❑ **SYRUP, DESSERT** *See* DESSERT SAUCES, SYRUPS, & TOPPINGS

❑ **TOFU, FROZEN** *See* DESSERTS, FROZEN

❑ **TREACLE** *See* SUGARS & SWEETENERS

❑ **TURKEY** *See* POULTRY, FRESH & PROCESSED; PROCESSED MEAT & POULTRY PRODUCTS

❑ **VEAL** *See* LAMB, VEAL, & MISCELLANEOUS MEATS

❑ **VEGETABLES, PLAIN & PREPARED**
See also LEGUMES & LEGUME PRODUCTS; PICKLES, OLIVES, RELISHES, & CHUTNEYS; RICE & GRAINS, PLAIN & PREPARED

Vegetables, Plain

amaranth					
raw	1 c	0	tr	tr	7
boiled, drained	½ c	0	tr	tr	14

	Portion	Chol (mg)	Total Fat (g)	Satur'd Fat (g)	Total Calor
arrowhead					
raw	1 medium corm = 0.4 oz	0	tr	?	12
boiled, drained	1 medium corm = 1.4 oz	0	tr	?	9
artichokes, globe & French varieties					
boiled	1 medium = 4.2 oz	0	tr	tr	53
	½ c hearts	0	tr	tr	37
frozen, boiled, drained	9 oz pkg	0	1	tr	108
artichokes, Jerusalem *See* Jerusalem artichokes, *below*					
asparagus, cuts & spears					
raw	4 spears = 2 oz	0	tr	tr	13
boiled	4 spears = 2.1 oz	0	tr	tr	15
canned					
drained solids	½ c	0	1	tr	24
solids & liquids	½ c	0	tr	tr	17
frozen, boiled, drained	10 oz pkg	0	1	tr	82
	4 spears = 2.1 oz	0	tr	tr	17
asparagus beans *See* yardlong beans, *under* LEGUMES & LEGUME PRODUCTS					
balsam pear					
leafy tips					
raw	½ c	0	tr	?	7
boiled, drained	½ c	0	tr	?	10
pods					
raw	1 c	0	tr	?	16
boiled, drained	½ c	0	tr	?	12
bamboo shoots					
raw	½ c	0	tr	tr	21
boiled, drained	1 c	0	tr	tr	15
canned, drained solids	1 c	0	1	tr	25
basella *See* vinespinach, *below*					
beans, shellie, canned, solids & liquids	½ c	0	tr	tr	37
beans, snap					
raw	½ c	0	tr	tr	17
boiled, drained	½ c	0	tr	tr	22
canned					
drained solids	½ c	0	tr	tr	13
solids & liquids	½ c	0	tr	tr	18
solids & liquids, seasoned	½ c	0	tr	tr	18
frozen, boiled, drained	½ c	0	tr	tr	18
beet greens					
raw	½ c	0	tr	tr	4
boiled, drained	½ c	0	tr	tr	20

	Portion	Chol (mg)	Total Fat (g)	Satur'd Fat (g)	Total Calor
beets					
raw	½ c sliced	0	tr	tr	30
boiled, drained	½ c sliced	0	tr	tr	26
canned					
drained solids	½ c sliced	0	tr	tr	27
solids & liquids	½ c sliced	0	tr	tr	36
pickled, canned, solids & liquids	½ c	0	tr	tr	75
beets, Harvard, canned, solids & liquids	½ c sliced	0	tr	tr	89
bittergourd; bittermelon *See* balsam pear, *above*					
bok choy *See* cabbage, Chinese, *below*					
borage					
raw	½ c	0	tr	?	9
boiled, drained	3½ oz	0	1	?	25
broad beans *See* LEGUMES & LEGUME PRODUCTS					
broccoli					
raw	1 spear = 5.3 oz	0	1	tr	42
boiled, drained	½ c	0	tr	tr	23
	1 spear = 6.3 oz	0	1	tr	53
frozen, boiled, drained	½ c chopped	0	tr	tr	25
	½ c spears	0	tr	tr	69
	10 oz pkg spears	0	tr	tr	25
brussels sprouts					
boiled, drained	1 sprout = 0.73 oz	0	tr	tr	8
	½ c	0	tr	tr	30
frozen, boiled, drained	½ c	0	tr	tr	33
burdock root					
raw	1 c	0	tr	?	85
	5½ oz	0	tr	?	112
boiled, drained	1 c	0	tr	?	110
	5.8 oz	0	tr	?	146
butterbur					
raw	1 c	0	tr	tr	13
boiled, drained	3½ oz	0	tr	tr	8
cabbage					
raw	½ c shredded	0	tr	tr	8
boiled, drained	½ c shredded	0	tr	tr	16
cabbage, Chinese					
bok choy					
raw	½ c shredded	0	tr	tr	5
boiled, drained	½ c shredded	0	tr	tr	10

	Portion	Chol (mg)	Total Fat (g)	Satur'd Fat (g)	Total Calor
cabbage, Chinese *(cont.)*					
pe-tsai					
raw	½ c shred-ded	0	tr	tr	6
boiled, drained	1 c shred-ded	0	tr	tr	16
cabbage, red					
raw	½ c shred-ded	0	tr	tr	10
boiled, drained	½ c shred-ded	0	tr	tr	16
cabbage, savoy					
raw	½ c shred-ded	0	tr	tr	10
boiled, drained	½ c shred-ded	0	tr	tr	18
cardoon, raw	½ c shred-ded	0	tr	tr	18
carrots					
raw	½ c shred-ded	0	tr	tr	24
	2½ oz	0	tr	tr	31
boiled, drained	½ c sliced	0	tr	tr	35
	1.6 oz	0	tr	tr	21
canned					
drained solids	½ c sliced	0	tr	tr	17
solids & liquids	½ c sliced	0	tr	tr	28
frozen, boiled, drained	½ c sliced	0	tr	tr	26
cassava, raw	3½ oz	0	tr	tr	120
cauliflower					
raw	½ c pieces	0	tr	tr	12
	3 flowerets = 2 oz	0	tr	tr	13
boiled, drained	½ c pieces	0	tr	tr	15
frozen, boiled, drained	½ c pieces	0	tr	tr	17
celeriac					
raw	½ c	0	tr	tr	31
boiled, drained	3½ oz	0	tr	?	25
celery					
raw	1 stalk = 1.4 oz	0	tr	tr	6
	½ c diced	0	tr	tr	9
boiled, drained	½ c diced	0	tr	tr	11
celtuce, raw	1 leaf = 0.3 oz	0	tr	?	2
chard, Swiss					
raw	½ c chopped	0	tr	?	3
boiled, drained	½ c chopped	0	tr	?	18

	Portion	Chol (mg)	Total Fat (g)	Satur'd Fat (g)	Total Calor
chayote, fruit					
raw	1 c pieces	0	tr	?	32
	7.1 oz	0	1	?	49
boiled, drained	1 c pieces	0	1	?	38
chicory, raw					
greens	½ c chopped	0	tr	tr	21
roots	½ c pieces	0	tr	tr	33
witloof	½ c	0	tr	tr	7
Chinese parsley *See* coriander, *below*					
Chinese preserving melon *See* wax gourd, *below*					
chives					
raw	1 t	0	tr	tr	0
	1 T	0	tr	tr	1
freeze-dried	1 T	0	tr	tr	1
chrysanthemum, garland					
raw	1 c pieces	0	tr	?	4
boiled, drained	½ c pieces	0	tr	?	10
collards					
raw	½ c chopped	0	tr	?	18
boiled, drained	½ c chopped	0	tr	?	13
frozen, boiled, drained	½ c chopped	0	tr	?	31
coriander (cilantro), raw	¼ c	0	tr	?	1
corn, sweet					
raw	½ c kernels	0	1	tr	66
	kernels from 1 ear	0	1	tr	77
boiled, drained	½ c kernels	0	1	tr	89
	kernels from 1 ear	0	1	tr	83
canned					
cream style	½ c	0	1	tr	93
in brine, drained solids	½ c	0	1	tr	66
in brine, solids & liquids	½ c	0	1	tr	79
vacuum pack	½ c	0	1	tr	83
w/red & green peppers, solids & liquids	½ c	0	1	tr	86
frozen, boiled, drained	½ c kernels	0	tr	tr	67
	kernels from 1 ear	0	tr	tr	59
cowpeas *See* LEGUMES & LEGUME PRODUCTS					
cress, garden					
raw	1 sprig	0	tr	0	0
	½ c	0	tr	tr	8
boiled, drained	½ c	0	tr	tr	16

	Portion	Chol (mg)	Total Fat (g)	Satur'd Fat (g)	Total Calor
cucumber, raw	½ c sliced	0	tr	tr	7
	10½ oz	0	tr	tr	39
daikon *See* radishes: Oriental, *below*					
dandelion greens					
raw	½ c chopped	0	tr	?	13
boiled, drained	½ c chopped	0	tr	?	17
dasheen *See* taro, *below*					
dock					
raw	½ c chopped	0	tr	?	15
boiled, drained	3½ oz	0	1	?	20
eggplant, boiled, drained	1 c cubed	0	tr	tr	27
endive, raw	½ c chopped	0	tr	tr	4
endive, Belgian *See* chickory: witloof, *above*					
eppaw, raw	½ c	0	1	?	75
escarole *See* endive, *above*					
garlic, raw	1 clove = 0.1 oz	0	tr	tr	4
ginger root, raw	0.4 oz	0	tr	tr	8
	¼ c sliced	0	tr	tr	17
gourd					
dishcloth, boiled, drained	½ c sliced	0	tr	tr	50
white-flowered (calabash), boiled, drained	½ c cubed	0	tr	tr	11
horseradish-tree					
leafy tips					
raw	½ c chopped	0	tr	?	6
boiled, drained	½ c chopped	0	tr	?	13
pods					
raw	1 pod = 0.4 oz	0	tr	?	4
boiled, drained	½ c sliced	0	tr	?	21
hyacinth beans *See* LEGUMES & LEGUME PRODUCTS					
Jerusalem artichokes, raw	½ c sliced	0	tr	0	57
jicama *See* yam bean, *below*					
jute (pot herb), boiled, drained	½ c	0	tr	tr	16
kale					
raw	½ c chopped	0	tr	tr	17
boiled, drained	½ c chopped	0	tr	tr	21
frozen, boiled, drained	½ c chopped	0	tr	tr	20
kale, Scotch					
raw	½ c chopped	0	tr	tr	14

	Portion	Chol (mg)	Total Fat (g)	Satur'd Fat (g)	Total Calor
boiled, drained	½ c chopped	0	tr	tr	18
kanpyo (dried gourd strips)	0.7 oz	0	tr	tr	49
kohlrabi					
raw	½ c sliced	0	tr	tr	19
boiled, drained	½ c sliced	0	tr	tr	24
lamb's-quarters, boiled, drained	½ c chopped	0	1	tr	29
leeks					
raw	¼ c chopped	0	tr	tr	16
boiled, drained	¼ c chopped	0	tr	tr	8
freeze-dried	1 T	0	0	0	1
lentils *See* LEGUMES & LEGUME PRODUCTS					
lettuce, raw					
butterhead (includes Boston & Bibb types)	2 leaves = ½ oz	0	tr	tr	2
	1 head = 5.7 oz	0	tr	tr	21
cos or romaine	1 inner leaf = 0.35 oz	0	tr	tr	2
	½ c shredded	0	tr	tr	4
iceberg	1 leaf = 0.7 oz	0	tr	tr	3
	1 head = 1 lb 3 oz	0	1	tr	70
looseleaf	1 leaf = 0.35 oz	0	tr	tr	2
	½ c shredded	0	tr	tr	5
lima beans *See* LEGUMES & LEGUME PRODUCTS					
lotus root, boiled, drained	3.1 oz	0	tr	tr	59
manioc *See* cassava, *above*					
mountain yam, Hawaii, steamed	½ c	0	tr	tr	59
mung beans *See* LEGUMES & LEGUME PRODUCTS					
mushrooms					
raw	½ c pieces	0	tr	tr	9
boiled, drained	½ c pieces	0	tr	tr	21
canned, drained solids	½ c pieces	0	tr	tr	19
mushrooms, shitake					
dried	0.1 oz	0	tr	tr	11
cooked	½ oz	0	tr	tr	40
mustard greens					
raw	½ c chopped	0	tr	tr	7
boiled, drained	½ c chopped	0	tr	tr	11

	Portion	Chol (mg)	Total Fat (g)	Satur'd Fat (g)	Total Calor
mustard greens *(cont.)*					
frozen, boiled, drained	½ c chopped	0	tr	tr	14
mustard spinach					
raw	½ c chopped	0	tr	?	17
boiled, drained	½ c chopped	0	tr	?	14
New Zealand spinach					
raw	½ c chopped	0	tr	tr	4
boiled, drained	½ c chopped	0	tr	tr	11
okra					
boiled, drained	½ c sliced	0	tr	tr	25
frozen, boiled, drained	½ c sliced	0	tr	tr	34
onions					
raw	1 T chopped	0	tr	tr	3
	½ c chopped	0	tr	tr	27
boiled, drained	1 T chopped	0	tr	tr	4
	½ c chopped	0	tr	tr	29
canned, solids & liquids	2.2 oz	0	tr	tr	12
dehydrated flakes	1 T	0	tr	tr	16
frozen, boiled, drained	1 T chopped	0	tr	tr	4
	½ c chopped	0	tr	tr	30
onions, spring, raw	1 T chopped	0	tr	tr	2
	½ c chopped	0	tr	tr	13
onions, Welsh, raw	3½ oz	0	tr	tr	34
oysterplant *See* salsify, *below*					
parsley					
raw	10 sprigs = 0.35 oz	0	tr	?	3
	½ c chopped	0	tr	?	10
freeze-dried	1 T	0	tr	?	1
parsnips					
raw	½ c sliced	0	tr	tr	50
boiled, drained	½ c sliced	0	tr	tr	63
peas, edible pods					
raw	½ c	0	tr	tr	30
boiled, drained	½ c	0	tr	tr	34
frozen, boiled, drained	½ c	0	tr	tr	42
	10 oz pkg	0	1	tr	132

	Portion	Chol (mg)	Total Fat (g)	Satur'd Fat (g)	Total Calor
peas, green					
raw	½ c	0	tr	tr	63
boiled, drained	½ c	0	tr	tr	67
canned					
drained solids	½ c	0	tr	tr	59
solids & liquids	½ c	0	tr	tr	61
solids & liquids, seasoned	½ c	0	tr	tr	57
frozen, boiled, drained	½ c	0	tr	tr	63
peas, mature seeds, sprouted					
raw	½ c	0	tr	tr	77
boiled, drained	3½ oz	0	1	tr	118
peas, split *See* split peas, *under* LEGUMES & LEGUME PRODUCTS					
peas & carrots					
canned, solids & liquids	½ c	0	tr	tr	48
frozen, boiled, drained	½ c	0	tr	tr	38
	10 oz pkg	0	1	tr	133
peas & onions					
canned, solids & liquids	½ c	0	tr	tr	30
frozen, boiled, drained	½ c	0	tr	tr	40
pepeao					
raw	0.2 oz	0	0	0	2
dried	½ c	0	tr	?	36
peppers					
hot chili					
raw	1 pepper = 1.6 oz	0	tr	tr	18
	½ c chopped	0	tr	tr	30
canned, solids & liquids	1 pepper = 2.6 oz	0	tr	tr	18
	½ c chopped	0	tr	tr	17
jalapeño, canned, solids & liquids	½ c chopped	0	tr	tr	17
sweet					
raw	1 pepper = 2.6 oz	0	tr	tr	18
	½ c chopped	0	tr	tr	12
boiled, drained	1 pepper = 2.6 oz	0	tr	tr	13
	½ c chopped	0	tr	tr	12
canned, solids & liquids	½ c halves	0	tr	tr	13
freeze-dried	1 T	0	tr	tr	1
	¼ c	0	tr	tr	5
frozen, unprepared, chopped	10 oz pkg	0	1	tr	58

	Portion	Chol (mg)	Total Fat (g)	Satur'd Fat (g)	Total Calor
peppers: sweet *(cont.)*					
frozen, boiled, drained	3½ oz chopped	0	tr	tr	18
pigeon peas *See* LEGUMES & LEGUME PRODUCTS					
pimientos *See* PICKLES, OLIVES, RELISHES, & CHUTNEYS					
pinto beans *See* LEGUMES & LEGUME PRODUCTS					
poi	½ c	0	tr	tr	134
pokeberry shoots					
raw	½ c	0	tr	?	18
boiled, drained	½ c	0	tr	?	16
potatoes					
raw					
flesh	3.9 oz	0	tr	tr	88
skin	1.3 oz	0	tr	tr	22
baked					
flesh & skin	7.1 oz	0	tr	tr	220
flesh	5½ oz	0	tr	tr	145
skin	2 oz	0	tr	tr	115
boiled in skin					
flesh	4.8 oz	0	tr	tr	119
skin	1.2 oz	0	tr	tr	27
boiled w/out skin, flesh	4.8 oz	0	tr	tr	116
canned					
drained solids	1.2 oz	0	tr	tr	21
solids & liquids	1 c	0	tr	tr	120
frozen, whole, unpre-pared	½ c	0	tr	tr	71
microwaved in skin					
flesh & skin	7.1 oz	0	tr	tr	212
flesh	5½ oz	0	tr	tr	156
skin	2 oz	0	tr	tr	77
pumpkin					
boiled, drained	½ c mashed	0	tr	tr	24
canned	½ c	0	tr	tr	41
pumpkin flowers					
raw	1 c	0	tr	tr	5
boiled, drained	½ c	0	tr	tr	10
pumpkin leaves, boiled, drained	½ c	0	tr	tr	7
purslane					
raw	1 c	0	tr	?	7
boiled, drained	1 c	0	tr	?	21
radishes, raw	10 radishes = 1.6 oz	0	tr	tr	7
Oriental					
raw	½ c	0	tr	tr	8
boiled, drained	½ c sliced	0	tr	tr	13
dried	½ c	0	tr	tr	157
white icicle, raw	½ c sliced	0	tr	tr	7
radish seeds, sprouted, raw	½ c	0	tr	tr	8

	Portion	Chol (mg)	Total Fat (g)	Satur'd Fat (g)	Total Calor
rutabagas					
raw	½ c cubed	0	tr	tr	25
boiled, drained	½ c cubed	0	tr	tr	29
	½ c mashed	0	tr	tr	41
salsify					
raw	½ c sliced	0	tr	?	55
boiled, drained	½ c sliced	0	tr	?	46
seaweed					
agar, raw	3½ oz	0	tr	tr	26
kelp, raw	3½ oz	0	1	tr	43
laver, raw	3½ oz	0	tr	tr	35
spirulina					
raw	3½ oz	0	tr	tr	26
dried	3½ oz	0	8	3	290
wakame, raw	3½ oz	0	1	tr	45
sesbania flower					
raw	1 c	0	tr	?	5
steamed	1 c	0	tr	?	23
shallots					
raw	1 T chopped	0	tr	tr	7
freeze-dried	1 T	0	tr	tr	3
snow peas See peas, edible pods, *above*					
soybeans See SOYBEANS & SOYBEAN PRODUCTS					
spinach					
raw	½ c chopped	0	tr	tr	6
boiled, drained	½ c	0	tr	tr	21
canned					
drained solids	½ c	0	1	tr	25
solids & liquids	½ c	0	tr	tr	22
frozen, boiled, drained	½ c	0	tr	tr	27
	10 oz pkg	0	tr	tr	63
spinach, mustard See mustard spinach, *above*					
spinach, New Zealand See New Zealand spinach, *above*					
split peas See LEGUMES & LEGUME PRODUCTS					
sprouts See *plant name (alfalfa, mung bean, etc.)*					
squash, summer					
all varieties					
raw	½ c sliced	0	tr	tr	13
boiled, drained	½ c sliced	0	tr	tr	18
crookneck					
raw	½ c sliced	0	tr	tr	12
boiled, drained	½ c sliced	0	tr	tr	18
canned, drained solids	½ c sliced	0	tr	tr	14
frozen, boiled, drained	½ c sliced	0	tr	tr	24
scallop					
raw	½ c sliced	0	tr	tr	12
boiled, drained	½ c sliced	0	tr	tr	14

	Portion	Chol (mg)	Total Fat (g)	Satur'd Fat (g)	Total Calor
squash, summer *(cont.)*					
zucchini					
raw	½ c sliced	0	tr	tr	9
boiled, drained	½ c sliced	0	tr	tr	14
canned, Italian style, in tomato sauce	½ c	0	tr	tr	33
frozen, boiled, drained	½ c	0	tr	tr	19
squash, winter					
all varieties					
raw	½ c cubed	0	tr	tr	21
baked	½ c cubed	0	1	tr	39
acorn					
baked	½ c cubed	0	tr	tr	57
boiled	½ c mashed	0	tr	tr	41
butternut					
baked	½ c cubed	0	tr	tr	41
frozen, boiled	½ c mashed	0	tr	tr	47
hubbard					
baked	½ c cubed	0	1	tr	51
boiled	½ c mashed	0	tr	tr	35
spaghetti, boiled, drained, baked	½ c	0	tr	tr	23
string beans *See* beans, snap, *above*					
succotash					
boiled, drained	½ c	0	1	tr	111
canned					
w/cream-style corn	½ c	0	1	tr	102
w/whole kernel corn, solids & liquids	½ c	0	1	tr	81
frozen, boiled, drained	½ c	0	1	tr	79
swamp cabbage					
raw	1 c chopped	0	tr	?	11
boiled, drained	1 c chopped	0	tr	?	20
sweet potatoes					
baked in skin	½ c mashed	0	tr	tr	103
	1 potato = 4 oz	0	tr	tr	118
boiled w/out skin	½ c mashed	0	tr	tr	172
candied	3.7 oz	8	3	1	144
canned					
in syrup, drained solids	1 c	0	1	tr	213
in syrup, solids & liquids	1 c	0	tr	tr	202

	Portion	Chol (mg)	Total Fat (g)	Satur'd Fat (g)	Total Calor
mashed	1 c	0	1	tr	258
vacuum packed	1 c pieces	0	tr	tr	183
	1 c mashed	0	1	tr	233
frozen, baked	½ c cubed	0	tr	tr	88
sweet potato leaves					
raw	1 c chopped	0	tr	tr	12
steamed	1 c	0	tr	tr	22
Swiss chard See chard, Swiss, above					
taro					
raw	½ c sliced	0	tr	tr	56
cooked	½ c sliced	0	tr	tr	94
taro chips	10 chips = 0.8 oz	0	6	2	110
taro leaves					
raw	1 c	0	tr	tr	12
steamed	1 c	0	1	tr	35
taro shoots					
raw	1 shoot = 2.9 oz	0	tr	tr	9
cooked	½ c sliced	0	tr	tr	10
taro, Tahitian					
raw	½ c sliced	0	1	tr	25
cooked	½ c sliced	0	tr	tr	30
tomatoes, green, raw	1 tomato = 4.3 oz	0	tr	tr	30
tomatoes, red, ripe					
raw	1 tomato = 4.3 oz	0	tr	tr	24
boiled	½ c	0	tr	tr	30
canned					
stewed	½ c	0	tr	tr	34
wedges in juice	½ c	0	tr	tr	34
w/green chilies	½ c	0	tr	tr	18
whole	½ c	0	tr	tr	24
stewed	1 c	0	2	tr	59
tomato paste, canned	½ c	0	1	tr	110
tomato puree, canned	1 c	0	tr	tr	102
tomato sauce See SAUCES, GRAVIES, & CONDIMENTS					
towel gourd See gourd: dishcloth, above					
tree fern, cooked	½ c chopped	?	tr	?	28
turnip greens					
raw	½ c chopped	0	tr	tr	7
boiled, drained	½ c chopped	0	tr	tr	15
canned, solids & liquids	½ c	0	tr	tr	17
frozen, boiled, drained	½ c	0	tr	tr	24
turnip greens & turnips, frozen, boiled, drained	3½ oz	0	tr	tr	17

	Portion	Chol (mg)	Total Fat (g)	Satur'd Fat (g)	Total Calor
turnips					
raw	½ c cubed	0	tr	tr	18
boiled, drained	½ c cubed	0	tr	tr	14
frozen, boiled, drained	3½ oz	0	tr	tr	23
vegetables, mixed					
canned					
drained solids	½ c	0	tr	tr	39
solids & liquids	½ c	0	tr	tr	44
frozen, boiled, drained	½ c	0	tr	tr	54
	10 oz pkg	0	tr	tr	163
vinespinach, raw	3½ oz	0	tr	?	19
water chestnuts, Chinese					
raw	1¼ oz	0	tr	?	38
canned, solids & liquids	1 oz	0	tr	?	14
watercress, raw	½ c chopped	0	tr	tr	2
wax beans See beans, snap, above					
wax gourd (Chinese pre-serving melon), boiled, drained	½ c cubed	0	tr	tr	11
winged beans See LEGUMES & LEGUME PRODUCTS					
yam, baked or boiled	½ c cubed	0	tr	tr	79
yam bean, tuber only					
raw	1 c sliced	0	tr	?	49
boiled, drained	3½ oz	0	tr	?	46
yardlong beans See LEGUMES & LEGUME PRODUCTS					

Vegetables, Prepared

	Portion	Chol (mg)	Total Fat (g)	Satur'd Fat (g)	Total Calor
coleslaw	½ c	5	2	tr	42
corn pudding	1 c	230	13	6	271
onion rings, breaded, frozen, heated in oven	0.7 oz	0	5	2	81
potato chips & sticks See SNACKS					
potatoes, au gratin					
dry mix, prepared	5½ oz pkg	?	34	21	764
homemade	½ c	29	9	6	160
potatoes, french-fried, frozen					
fried in animal fat & vegetable oil	1.8 oz	6	8	3	158
fried in vegetable oil	1.8 oz	0	8	3	158
heated in oven	1.8 oz	0	4	2	111
cottage-cut, heated in oven	1.8 oz	0	4	2	109
extruded, heated in oven	1.8 oz	0	9	4	163
potatoes, hashed brown					
frozen, plain, prepared	½ c	?	9	4	170
frozen, w/butter sauce, unprepared	6 oz pkg	?	11	4	229

	Portion	Chol (mg)	Total Fat (g)	Satur'd Fat (g)	Total Calor
homemade, prepared in vegetable oil	½ c	?	11	4	163
potatoes, mashed					
dehydrated flakes, prepared (whole milk & butter added)	½ c	15	6	4	118
granules w/milk, prepared	½ c	2	2	1	83
granules w/out milk, prepared (whole milk & butter added)	½ c	18	7	1	137
homemade w/whole milk & margarine	½ c	2	4	1	111
homemade w/whole milk	½ c	2	1	tr	81
potatoes, O'Brien					
frozen, prepared	3½ oz	?	13	3	204
homemade	1 c	7	2	2	157
potatoes, scalloped					
dry mix, prepared w/ whole milk & butter	5½ oz pkg	?	35	22	764
homemade	½ c	14	4	3	105
potato flour *See* FLOURS & CORNMEALS					
potato pancakes, homemade	2.7 oz	93	13	3	495
potato puffs, frozen, fried in vegetable oil	¼ oz	0	1	tr	16
potato salad	½ c	86	10	2	179
sauerkraut, canned, solids & liquids	½ c	0	tr	tr	22
spinach soufflé	1 c	184	18	7	218

▪ BRAND NAME

Arrowhead Mills

potato flakes	2 oz	0	0	?	140

Birds Eye Frozen Vegetables.

all Regular, Deluxe, & Farm Fresh frozen vegetables	1 serving	0	0–1	0–1	varies

CHEESE SAUCE COMBINATION

baby brussels sprouts w/ cheese sauce	4½ oz	5	6	?	110
broccoli w/cheese sauce	5 oz	5	6	?	120
broccoli w/creamy Italian cheese sauce	4½ oz	15	6	?	90
cauliflower w/cheese sauce	5 oz	5	6	?	110

	Portion	Chol (mg)	Total Fat (g)	Satur'd Fat (g)	Total Calor
peas & pearl onions w/ cheese sauce	5 oz	5	5	?	140

COMBINATION

broccoli, carrots, pasta twists	3.3 oz	0	4	?	90
corn, green beans, pasta curls	3.3 oz	0	5	?	110
creamed spinach	3 oz	0	4	?	60
fresh green beans w/ toasted almonds	3 oz	0	2	?	50
green peas & pearl onions	3.3 oz	0	0	0	70
green peas & potatoes w/ cream sauce	2.6 oz	0	6	?	130
mixed vegetables w/onion sauce	2.6 oz	0	5	?	100
rice & green peas w/mush-rooms	2.3 oz	0	0	0	110
small onions w/cream sauce	3 oz	0	6	?	110

INTERNATIONAL RECIPES

Bavarian style	3.3 oz	10	6	?	110
Chinese style	3.3 oz	0	5	?	80
chow mein style	3.3 oz	0	4	?	90
Italian style	3.3 oz	0	7	?	110
Japanese style	3.3 oz	0	6	?	100
Mandarin style	3.3 oz	0	4	?	90
New England style	3.3 oz	0	7	?	130
pasta primavera style	3.3 oz	5	5	?	120
San Francisco style	3.3 oz	0	5	?	100

STIR-FRY

Chinese style	3.3 oz	0	0	0	35
Japanese style	3.3 oz	0	0	0	30
Chun King					
bamboo shoots	2 oz	?	0	?	16
bean sprouts	4 oz	?	0	?	40
chow mein vegetables	4 oz	?	0	?	35
water chestnuts, whole, sliced	2 oz	?	0	?	45
Claussen					
sauerkraut	½ c	?	tr	tr	17
Fresh Chef					
Holiday cole slaw	4 oz	?	15	?	200
Old Fashioned potato salad	4 oz	?	14	?	210
Joan of Arc					
all canned vegetables	½ c	?	<10	?	varies

	Portion	Chol (mg)	Total Fat (g)	Satur'd Fat (g)	Total Calor
Mrs. Paul's Prepared Vegetables					
candied yams	4 oz	?	1	?	200
corn fritters	2	?	12	?	250
eggplant parmigiana	5½ oz	?	17	?	270
fried eggplant sticks	3½ oz	?	12	?	240
onion rings, crispy	2½ oz	?	10	?	180
zucchini sticks, light batter	3 oz	?	12	?	200
Ortega					
green chiles, whole, diced, strips, sliced	1 oz	?	0	?	10
hot peppers, whole, diced	1 oz	?	0	?	8
jalapeño peppers, whole, diced	1 oz	?	0	?	10
tomatoes & jalapeños	1 oz	?	0	?	8
Pepperidge Farm Vegetables in Pastry					
broccoli w/cheese	1	?	17	?	250
cauliflower & cheese sauce	1	?	13	?	210
Pillsbury					
all canned vegetables	½ c	?	<10	?	varies
all Butter Sauce & Cream & Cheese Sauce Combination frozen vegetables	½ c	?	<6	?	varies
all Harvest Get Togethers, Harvest Fresh, Polybag, & Valley Combination Dual Pouch frozen vegetables	½ c	?	<6	?	varies
stuffed baked potato w/ cheese-flavored topping	1	?	6	?	200
stuffed baked potato w/ sour cream & chives	1	?	10	?	230
Stouffer					
broccoli in cheddar cheese sauce	4½ oz	?	10	?	150
corn soufflé	4 oz	?	7	?	150
creamed spinach	4½ oz	?	15	?	190
green bean mushroom casserole	4¾ oz	?	12	?	170
potatoes au gratin	⅓ of 11½ oz pkg	?	6	?	120
scalloped potatoes	4 oz	?	6	?	110
spinach soufflé	4 oz	?	9	?	140
yams & apples	5 oz	?	3	?	160

	Portion	Chol (mg)	Total Fat (g)	Satur'd Fat (g)	Total Calor
Vlasic					
Old Fashioned sauerkraut	1 oz	0	0	0	4

❑ **VINEGAR** *See* SALAD DRESSINGS, MAYONNAISE, VINEGAR, & DIPS

❑ **WHEY** *See* MILK, MILK SUBSTITUTES, & MILK PRODUCTS

❑ **YOGURT** *See* MILK, MILK SUBSTITUTES, & MILK PRODUCTS

❑ **YOGURT, FROZEN** *See* DESSERTS, FROZEN